NATIONAL ACADEMIES
Sciences
Engineering
Medicine

NATIONAL
ACADEMIES
PRESS
Washington, DC

AF395542

Exploring the Treatment and Management of Chronic Pain and Implications for Disability Determinations

Convened April 17–18, 2025

Austen Applegate, Rebecca A. English, and Joe Alper, *Rapporteurs*

Board on Health Care Services

Health and Medicine Division

Proceedings of a Workshop

NATIONAL ACADEMIES PRESS 500 Fifth Street, NW Washington, DC 20001

This activity was supported by contracts between the National Academy of Sciences and the U.S. Social Security Administration (Contract #28321323D00060012/Task Order #28321324FDS030149). Any opinions, findings, conclusions, or recommendations expressed in this publication do not necessarily reflect the views of any organization or agency that provided support for the project.

International Standard Book Number-13: 978-0-309-99513-9
Digital Object Identifier: https://doi.org/10.17226/29181

This publication is available from the National Academies Press, 500 Fifth Street, NW, Keck 360, Washington, DC 20001; (800) 624-6242; http://www.nap.edu.

The manufacturer's authorized representative in the European Union for product safety is Authorised Rep Compliance Ltd., Ground Floor, 71 Lower Baggot Street, Dublin D02 P593 Ireland; www.arccompliance.com.

Suggested citation: National Academies of Sciences, Engineering, and Medicine. 2025. *Exploring the treatment and management of chronic pain and implications for disability determinations: Proceedings of a workshop.* Washington, DC: National Academies Press. https://doi.org/10.17226/29181.

The **National Academy of Sciences** was established in 1863 by an Act of Congress, signed by President Lincoln, as a private, nongovernmental institution to advise the nation on issues related to science and technology. Members are elected by their peers for outstanding contributions to research. Dr. Marcia McNutt is president.

The **National Academy of Engineering** was established in 1964 under the charter of the National Academy of Sciences to bring the practices of engineering to advising the nation. Members are elected by their peers for extraordinary contributions to engineering. Dr. Tsu-Jae Liu is president.

The **National Academy of Medicine** (formerly the Institute of Medicine) was established in 1970 under the charter of the National Academy of Sciences to advise the nation on medical and health issues. Members are elected by their peers for distinguished contributions to medicine and health. Dr. Victor J. Dzau is president.

The three Academies work together as the **National Academies of Sciences, Engineering, and Medicine** to provide independent, objective analysis and advice to the nation and conduct other activities to solve complex problems and inform public policy decisions. The National Academies also encourage education and research, recognize outstanding contributions to knowledge, and increase public understanding in matters of science, engineering, and medicine.

Learn more about the National Academies of Sciences, Engineering, and Medicine at **www.nationalacademies.org**.

**PLANNING COMMITTEE ON EXPLORING THE
TREATMENT AND MANAGEMENT OF CHRONIC PAIN
AND IMPLICATIONS FOR DISABILITY DETERMINATION[1]**

ALLEN HEINEMANN (*Chair*), Northwestern University
TAMARA BAKER, University of North Carolina at Chapel Hill
ANIRBAN BASU, University of Washington
REUBEN ESCORPIZO, University of Vermont
JUAN HINCAPIE-CASTILLO, University of North Carolina at Chapel
 Hill
KIM DUPREE JONES, Emory University
SEAN MACKEY, Stanford Medical School
CHRISTOPHER STANDAERT, University of Pittsburgh
ANNA WILLIAMS, Clusterbusters
HENRY XIANG, The Ohio State University and Nationwide Children's
 Hospital

Project Staff

REBECCA A. ENGLISH, Senior Program Officer
AUSTEN APPLEGATE, Research Associate
ELIANA PIEROTTI, Senior Program Assistant
SHARYL NASS, Senior Director, Board on Health Care Services

National Academy of Medicine Fellow

SEBASTIAN TONG, University of Washington

Consultant

JOE ALPER, Science Writer

---

v

Reviewers

This Proceedings of a Workshop was reviewed in draft form by individuals chosen for their diverse perspectives and technical expertise. The purpose of this independent review is to provide candid and critical comments that will assist the National Academies of Sciences, Engineering, and Medicine in making each published proceedings as sound as possible and to ensure that it meets the institutional standards for quality, objectivity, evidence, and responsiveness to the charge. The review comments and draft manuscript remain confidential to protect the integrity of the process.

We thank the following individuals for their review of this proceedings:

SHRAVANI DURBHAKULA, Vanderbilt University Medical Center
LAURA SIMONS, Stanford Medical School
ANNA WILLIAMS, Clusterbusters

Although the reviewers listed above provided many constructive comments and suggestions, they were not asked to endorse the content of the proceedings nor did they see the final draft before its release. The review of this proceedings was overseen by **CLARION JOHNSON,** ExxonMobil (Ret.). He was responsible for making certain that an independent examination of this proceedings was carried out in accordance with standards of the National Academies and that all review comments were carefully considered. We also thank National Academies staff member Anthony Janifer for reading and providing helpful comments on this manuscript. Responsibility for the final content rests entirely with the rapporteurs and the National Academies.

Acknowledgments

The National Academies of Sciences, Engineering, and Medicine wish to thank all the members of the planning committee, who collaborated to ensure a workshop replete with informative presentations and moderated rich discussions, as well as the speakers, who generously shared their expertise and their time with workshop participants. Funding from the Social Security Administration made this workshop possible.

Contents

Boxes, Figures, and Table

TABLE

Acronyms and Abbreviations

ACT	acceptance and commitment therapy
CBT	cognitive behavioral therapy
CIPM	complementary and integrative pain management
EHR	electronic health record
FDA	Food and Drug Administration
FQHC	federally qualified health center
GET	graded exposure treatment
MBSR	mindfulness-based stress reduction
NLP	natural language processing
RA	rheumatoid arthritis
SGA	substantial gainful activity
SSA	Social Security Administration
TCQ	tai chi/qigong
VA	Veterans Administration

1

Introduction[1]

Chronic pain, defined as pain that persists for more than three months, is a pervasive and debilitating condition that can significantly affect a person's ability to work and function, potentially leading to disability.[2] Understanding the relationship between chronic pain and disability is crucial for developing effective management strategies and improving the quality of life for those affected.

The Social Security Administration (SSA) administers two programs that provide cash payments to people with disabilities: the Social Security Disability Insurance program and the Supplemental Security Income program. Social Security Disability Insurance, a program for workers who contribute through payroll tax deductions, aims to protect those workers from lost earnings arising because of impairment, while Supplemental

---

[1] The planning committee's role was limited to planning the workshop, and the Proceedings of a Workshop has been prepared by the workshop rapporteurs as a factual summary of what occurred at the workshop. Statements, recommendations, and opinions expressed are those of individual presenters and participants, and are not necessarily endorsed or verified by the National Academies of Sciences, Engineering, and Medicine, and they should not be construed as reflecting any group consensus.

[2] The International Association for the Study of Pain defines chronic pain as pain that persists for longer than 3 months. This type of pain often becomes the sole or predominant clinical problem in some patients. As such it may warrant specific diagnostic evaluation, therapy, and rehabilitation. Chronic pain is a frequent condition, affecting an estimated 20 percent of people worldwide, and is multifactorial—biological, psychological, and social factors contribute to the pain syndrome. https://www.iasp-pain.org/advocacy/definitions-of-chronic-pain-syndromes/ (accessed June 17, 2025).

Security Income's goal is to guarantee a base income for low-income people with disabilities and older adults.

To better understand the effects of chronic pain, how it is treated and managed, and its implications for disability determination, the Health and Medicine Division of the National Academies of Sciences, Engineering, and Medicine hosted a one-and-a-half-day workshop on April 17–18, 2025, that explored the many experiences and challenges related to chronic pain and its management, and how these experiences affect health status, functional limitations, and medical records for both children and adults. Box 1-1 provides the statement of task for the workshop, which SSA funded.

Robert Weathers, deputy associate commissioner for SSA's Office of Disability Policy, noted in his introductory remarks to the workshop that accurately evaluating a disability claim has "been a thorn in the side of SSA adjudicators since the administration first began paying disability benefits nearly 70 years ago." The challenge with chronic pain is that it is a wholly individualized experience, and there is no objective test or laboratory value that SSA can rely on to understand the extent to which chronic pain is interfering with an individual's ability to work and function. That said, SSA has set policies and existing guidance on pain evaluation that it provides to its adjudicators, but Weathers asked the workshop participants to consider how SSA can give its adjudicators a better understanding of and more actionable guidance on pain evaluation while maintaining the essential flexibility and latitude needed to guide people through a uniform disability determination process.

This Proceedings of a Workshop summarizes the presentations and discussions, reflecting the speakers', panelists', and participants' broad range of views and ideas. The speakers' presentations (as PDFs and video files) are available online.[3]

---

[3] https://www.nationalacademies.org/event/43975_04-2025_exploring-the-treatment-and-management-of-chronic-pain-and-implications-for-disability-determinations-a-workshop (accessed July 24, 2025).

BOX 1-1
Statement of Task

A planning committee of the National Academies of Sciences, Engineering, and Medicine will organize and host a 1 to 2 day public workshop to explore the wide variety of experiences and challenges related to chronic pain and its management. The workshop will include presentations with a focus on how those different experiences impact an individual's health status, functional limitations, and medical records.

The workshop will feature invited presentations and panel discussions on topics such as:

- Current best practices and professional philosophy for the management of individuals' chronic pain;
- Methods of categorization for chronic pain and the salient factors that identify individuals' pain as falling within particular categories;
- Recent advancements and promising developments in the measurement of chronic pain levels;
- Special considerations in how medical providers approach treatment of chronic pain with varying or episodic severity compared to pain with relatively constant severity;
- Special considerations or challenges for medical providers in the management of chronic pain in children;
- Alternative and complementary pain treatments pursued by individuals experiencing chronic pain, the efficacy of those treatments, how they may be reflected in the medical record, and implications for, or interactions with, traditional treatment paradigms;
- The lived experiences of people with chronic pain as they seek medical care and navigate the SSA disability system; and
- An overview of recent or emerging research on new or improved methods for the measurement and management on chronic pain.

The planning committee will develop the agenda for the workshop sessions, select and invite speakers and discussants, and moderate the discussions. A proceedings of the presentations and discussions at the workshop will be prepared by a designated rapporteur in accordance with institutional guidelines.

2

Overview, Concepts, and Framing of Chronic Pain and Disability

The workshop opened with a high-level overview of topics that served as background for the remainder of the workshop. The three speakers were Vincent Nibali, a technical expert in the Social Security Administration's (SSA's) Office of Medical Policy; Kim Dupree Jones, the Asa Griggs Chandler professor and associate dean for academic advancement at Emory University; and Jerome Bickenbach, permanent visiting professor at the University of Lucerne and professor emeritus at Queen's University, Canada.

DISABILITY ADJUDICATION POLICY

Vincent Nibali summarized SSA's disability adjudication process and how chronic pain can fit into that process. He explained that while SSA's two disability-related programs are designed for distinct populations, the medical and vocational rules for the two programs are identical once SSA determines an individual meets the non medical eligibility requirements for either program. He noted that both programs are for individuals who are totally disabled, an admittedly high standard whose purpose is to ensure benefits for those with long-term, disabling conditions.

For the purposes of determining program eligibility, Congress has defined disability for an adult as "the inability to engage in any substantial gainful activity (SGA) because of a medically determinable physical or mental impairment(s) that can be expected to result in death or that has lasted or that can be expected to last for a continuous period of not less than 12 months." SGA, said Nibali, is defined by a monetary amount. In

2025 SGA is considered earnings of $1,620 or more per month for most disabled people, or $2,700 per month for blind individuals.

For children, Congress has defined disability as "a medically determinable physical or mental impairment or combination of impairments that causes marked and severe functional limitations, and that can be expected to result in death or that has lasted or can be expected to last for a continuous period of not less than 12 months. An impairment(s) causes marked and severe functional limitations if it meets or medically equals the severity of a set of criteria for an impairment in the listings, or if it functionally equals the listings." The listings of impairments are special rules that help SSA identify claims that clearly meet the definition of disability (see Box 2-1).

To determine if an adult meets the requirement to be unable to engage in SGA, SSA has a five-question, sequential evaluation that allows it to make a disability decision at the earliest possible step without prejudicing any claimants:

1. Is the individual engaged in SGA?
2. Is the impairment a medically determinable physical or mental impairment that is severe, and does it meet the duration requirement?
3. Does the individual's medical condition meet or medically equal a listing, where listings are publicly available sets of criteria for specific impairments that SSA believes represent a higher level of limitation than the program requires in general?
4. Does the impairment prevent the individual from performing their past relevant work?
5. Does the individual have the ability to adjust to other work?

BOX 2-1
Listings of Impairments

Listings of impairments describe for each of the major body systems impairments that SSA considers to be severe enough to prevent an individual from doing any gainful activity, regardless of age, education, or work experience. In the case of children under age 18, the impairment must be severe enough to cause marked and severe functional limitations. The listings are special rules that provide SSA with a mechanism to identify clearly eligible claims. An impairment (or combination of impairments) is medically equal to an impairment in the listings if it is at least equal in severity and duration to the criteria of any listed impairment.

SOURCE: Nibali presentation, April 17, 2025.

Nibali explained that step 3 is a "screen-in" step, meaning if an individual does not qualify for disability benefits at this step, they are not denied, and the assessment moves to step 4. If an impairment is severe but does not meet or medically equal any listing, SSA assesses in step 4 whether the applicant's physical or mental residual functional capacity allows the person to perform past relevant work. Applicants who are able to perform past relevant work are denied benefits, while those who are unable to do so proceed to step 5. At step 5, SSA considers an applicant's residual functional capacity along with vocational factors such as age, education, and work experience, including transferable skills, in determining whether the individual can perform other work. Applicants determined to be unable to adjust to performing other work are allowed benefits, while those determined able to adjust are denied.

For children, SSA follows the first two steps in the adult process, but at step 3, after considering whether an impairment meets or medically equals the requirements of a listing, SSA additionally relies on the concept of "functionally equaling the listings,"[1] which means that an impairment must result in marked limitations in two domains of functioning or an extreme limitation in one domain compared to children of the same age without impairments. The six domains of functioning are acquiring and using information, attending and completing tasks, interacting and relating with others, moving about and manipulating objects, caring for oneself, and health and physical well-being.

Given there is no objective test or laboratory value to quantify pain itself as a severe, medically determinable physical or mental impairment as required by step 2, Nibali said SSA considers the extent to which an individual's symptoms, including pain, can be reasonably accepted as consistent with the objective medical evidence and other evidence, including the individual's statements and information from both medical and nonmedical sources. The key, he said, is consistency across all information sources. SSA tells its adjudicators to recognize that some individuals experience symptoms and related functional limitations differently, even with the same impairment and even with the same or similar case evidence. "I think that is essential because it speaks to the individual nature of chronic pain and the fact that we are not going to be able to look at a number on a page and make a decision," Nibali said.

CHRONIC PAIN TREATMENT

Kim Dupree Jones said research has shown that pain is not merely a symptom of injury or illness but is a disease entity that can become

---

[1] CFR § 416.926a.

self-perpetuating. She noted it takes an average of two to three years and seeing three to four physicians before an individual receives a diagnosis of certain pain conditions. This delay may be associated with poorer outcomes, including worsening severity (Choy et al., 2010; Clauw et al., 2019; Moshrif et al., 2023; Salaffi et al., 2024).

Jones said one challenge leading to a delay in diagnosing and treating pain is that many painful conditions overlap, making it difficult for a primary care physician to decide who to refer the patient to for further evaluation and treatment (Figure 2-1; Maixner et al., 2016; Schirle et al., 2023; Schrepf et al., 2024). Pain is not a stand-alone problem but one that exists with other symptoms, which often results in functional impairment. Difficulty standing or sitting for any length of time can accompany pain, as can fatigue, non-refreshing sleep, stiffness, tenderness to touch, and poor balance and falls related to postural limitations (Jones et al., 2011).

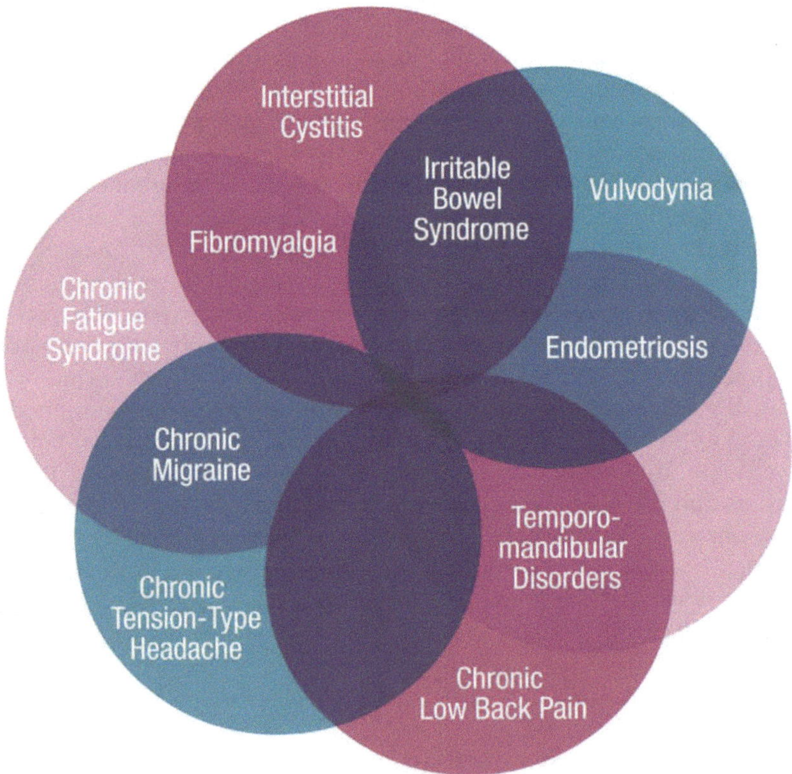

FIGURE 2-1 Overlap of many painful conditions.
SOURCE: Jones presentation, April 17, 2025; Chronic Pain Research Alliance, 2023. ©2023 Chronic Pain Research Alliance, An Initiative of The TMJ Association, Ltd. All rights reserved; used with permission.

Behavioral co-occurring symptoms can include depression, anxiety, and cognitive issues, including difficulty with short-term recall, sustained concentration, maintaining attention, and refocusing after distraction.

Symptoms can also flare after exertion (Barhorst et al., 2021). Jones, for example, has had patients repeatedly lift a 10-pound weight or go up and down stairs without trouble as part of a disability evaluation only to have a terrible delayed-onset symptom flare two or three days later. "I am not sure how we get around that, because they can generally rise to the occasion to do the task but then have an issue after that task is over," she noted.

Sensitivity to bright light (Balba et al., 2022), loud noises, cold, and odors are important co-occurring symptoms, said Jones. This is particularly true for nociplastic pain states that arise because of changes in how the nervous system processes pain signals and are associated with fibromyalgia, chronic low back pain, and irritable bowel syndrome. This has implications for how employers can make accommodations to keep people in the workplace.

Jones noted that pain diagnosis and treatment may be different in children and adolescents. It is important, she added, for children and adolescents not to fall through the cracks when they transition from pediatric to adult care.

Jones said there are opportunities to improve pain education for nurses and other health care providers to address the fact that the incidence of chronic pain is too high to be managed only in specialty care or pain clinics. "There is evidence that faculty do not really understand the relationship between acute pain moving to chronic pain and regional pain moving to widespread pain," said Jones (Firestone et al., 2025). It is important, too, she added, to listen to people with lived experience of chronic pain (Friend et al., 2021).

THE SOCIAL EVOLUTION OF CHRONIC PAIN

Jerome Bickenbach noted there are social policies, such as the benefits associated with Social Security disability determination, workers' compensation, and veteran status, that influence the social response to people who experience pain. Increasingly, these policies encourage people to maintain their employment and companies to introduce accommodations to keep people employed. Unlike the United States, however, most countries do not require the person to be totally unable to work in order to receive disability benefits.

Bickenbach said the driver of shifts in social conceptions of chronic pain is the unavoidable fact that pain is subjective. This subjective nature, in the context of disability determination, can raise suspicion of fraud and deception in self-reports of pain. He noted the conflation of impairment and disability or disease is at the center of the rules and regulations pertaining to disability determination. He pointed out that even if social policy recognized pain as a disability or as a disease, as opposed to a symptom of a disease or an impairment, practical issues would remain regarding the evidence of pain, the political acceptability of trusting self-report, and levels of individual sensitivity or cultural differences that may unfairly distort an assessment of pain severity and an individual's need for support.

3

Factors Affecting Access to Effective Chronic Pain Care

In the workshop's first session, participants considered the lived experiences of people with chronic pain as they seek medical care, discussed the variety of experiences and challenges related to managing chronic pain, and explored how variations in access to chronic pain interventions can affect the care individuals receive and the health care outcomes they experience. The three speakers were Jaime Sanders, author and patient advocate; Edwin Aroke, associate professor and assistant dean for research and scholarship at the University of Alabama at Birmingham School of Nursing; and Staja Booker, assistant professor at the University of Florida College of Nursing.

LIVING WITH MIGRAINE

Jaime Sanders said she has experienced chronic pain from migraine disease for most of her life, with her first migraine attack occurring when she was eight years old. Her mother's family has a history of migraine, but she was told by most of her physicians that she would outgrow it by the time she turned 18. That did not turn out to be the case; she experienced as many as eight migraines a month throughout her early 20s. In 2001, during the first trimester of a pregnancy, she experienced her first intractable migraine, which did not resolve until her second trimester. Her migraines did not stop, though, and became more severe and frequent. Sanders likened living with chronic migraine to navigating a minefield and never knowing when the next pain explosion will come.

Migraine is a debilitating and pervasive disorder affecting every facet of life, said Sanders. It is frequently misunderstood, trivialized, and dismissed as merely a bad headache. This dismissal is challenging for those who suffer from migraine, she added, as they are constantly forced to validate their pain. "The struggle of living with an 'invisible illness' like migraine begins with the simple fact that others cannot see your pain," she said. "This lack of visibility can lead to misunderstanding, skepticism, and even outright disbelief. It can make you feel as though your experience is invalid or exaggerated; that the agony you endure is somehow less real because it cannot be easily observed."

The invisible nature of migraine and other forms of chronic pain extends beyond physical symptoms to the emotional and psychological toll they take, creating a complex web of challenges that others often disregard. "I think there is a disconnect between the physical and emotional aspect of chronic pain, and they are not always treated together," said Sanders. She noted that migraine is a debilitating neurological condition with a broad range of symptoms, and finding effective treatment is challenging, despite its prevalence.

The lack of effective treatment options for migraine and chronic pain is a major issue for the millions of people living with these conditions, said Sanders. While there have been advances, many people struggle to find treatments that work for them or that they can afford, given the high costs associated with migraine treatments. As part of her advocacy work, Sanders has emphasized the need for more research funding and policy changes that would expand insurance coverage and eliminate copays for diagnostic procedures and migraine treatments, particularly newer, more effective medications. There is also a need, she said, to establish and expand financial assistance programs that provide direct financial support to migraine patients who cannot afford the high cost of treatment.

Sanders said that for her as a Black woman, the "intersection of race, gender, and chronic illness has been a central part" of her experience, influencing how health care providers have perceived and treated her, how she navigates social and professional spaces, and how she understands and manages her own health. She added that disparities in access, treatment quality, and outcomes for people of color, and particularly Black women, can significantly affect the experience of chronic illness. Studies have shown, for example, that Black patients are less likely to receive adequate pain management compared to White patients presenting with the same symptoms (Hoffman et al., 2016; Knoebel et al., 2021). Migraine, she added, is often seen as a "women's disease," partly because it affects women at three times the rate of men. As a result, it is sometimes dismissed as being hormonal or psychosomatic rather than recognized as a serious neurological disorder. "This can lead to a lack of understanding and empathy from health care providers as well as from friends, family members, and employers," she said.

When health care providers fail to take patients' pain seriously, they are less likely to prescribe effective treatments, less likely to refer patients to specialists, and less likely to provide the comprehensive care needed to manage a chronic condition, Sanders explained.

BIOLOGICAL MECHANISMS OF SOCIALLY DETERMINED PAIN AND THE IMPLICATIONS FOR PAIN MANAGEMENT

Edwin Aroke said a wide set of nonmedical forces and systems, such as economic and social policies and systems, shapes daily life and influences outcomes for people with chronic pain. These social factors, which he called the "social determinants of pain," include an individual's economic stability, access to quality education, access to quality health care, neighborhood and built environment, and social and community context. These factors can account for significant variations in health outcomes (Kapos et al., 2024), he said.

Aroke said that epigenetic changes[1] could be the link between the social and biological factors involved in chronic pain (Aroke et al., 2019). He explained that early experiences and environmental exposures can have lifelong and transgenerational effects via epigenetic changes, which regulate how genes are turned on and off at different times, thereby predisposing some people to experience non-specific chronic low back pain. Aroke and colleagues (2022a) found that epigenetic stressors—such as stigma, discrimination, and social injustice—disproportionately affecting Black individuals can lead to epigenetic modifications that heighten the risk of developing non-specific chronic low back pain. It has also been demonstrated that internalized stigma of chronic pain is associated with both worse pain outcomes and epigenetic changes in a signaling pathway that plays a prominent role in stress regulation (Aroke et al., 2022b).

Biological age, which is accelerated by chronic stress, may be another factor involved in determining who is more likely to develop chronic pain. For example, when he and his colleagues estimated an individual's biological age from their DNA, they found that biological aging was a stronger predictor of chronic pain than chronological age and that the acceleration of biological aging was worse for Black individuals compared to White individuals (Freij et al., 2024). One implication of these findings is that shared exposures to social determinants of pain are root causes of pain disparities, said Aroke. Social and structural forces not only affect treatment outcomes

---

[1] Epigenetic changes are defined as "a mechanism by which environmental factors such as childhood stress, racial discrimination, economic hardship, and depression can affect gene expression without altering the underlying genetic sequence" (Aroke et al., 2019).

but also mediate epigenetic and nervous system changes that sustain pain disparities across lifetimes, generations, and cultural histories.

CHRONIC PAIN, DISABILITY, AND AGING ACROSS IDENTITIES

Staja Booker reiterated that chronic pain is not a singular syndrome or disease but a multisystem disease. She also stressed that chronic pain is a disease state, not a symptom, and that disability results from a trajectory of disablement rather than a single cause. It is important, she said, to consider how chronic pain affects cognition and contributes to frailty and mortality, and she added that timely disability determination is important for effectively managing chronic pain.

According to the 2023 National Health Interview Survey, an estimated 21 million Americans have high-impact chronic pain that significantly restricts a person's daily activities and ability to function. Booker noted the prevalence of high-impact chronic pain increases with age. While experiencing pain at some point in life may be universal, for some people, pain is incurable and disabling, causing physical and psychological limitations and challenges. The invisible nature of pain contributes to disparities, said Booker, and within the last decade, there have been efforts to create more equitable pain care solutions through research. She stressed the need to ensure that "all with chronic pain have timely access and equal and personalized treatment," she said.

Recent research on differences in pain and disability among Black and White individuals with osteoarthritis has found that Black people experience significantly greater chronic pain and disability and worse scores on a short physical performance battery (Bartley et al., 2019; Vaughn et al., 2019). Booker and her collaborators have also studied pain trajectories and found that younger, less-educated, lower-income, and non-Hispanic Black study participants with knee osteoarthritis had greater representation in the highest pain trajectory group and were missing from the low pain trajectory group, while White adults fell largely into the low and moderate-low pain trajectory categories (Johnson et al., 2021). This suggests that Black adults start at a disadvantage in developing knee osteoarthritis. Family support, she added, can also affect the development of chronic pain in older Black adults (Woods et al., 2024).

Booker explained that pain-affirming care is a nonjudgmental approach that goes beyond accepting and believing patients' reports of pain. It validates their lived experience of pain and manages pain using timely, personalized strategies based on evidence while ensuring the individual understands the treatments that are available (Booker and Okolie, 2024).

4

Methods and Metrics for Chronic Pain Assessment in Adults and Children

The workshop's second session discussed best practices and methods of categorization for chronic pain; advances in treating, managing, and measuring chronic pain levels in children and adults; and how the assessment of chronic pain connects to assessments of function, performance, behavior, and disability. The four speakers were Deb Constien, a person with lived chronic pain experience; Steven George, the Laszlo Ormandy Distinguished Professor of orthopedic surgery at Duke University; Carole Tucker, professor and associate dean of research at the University of Texas Medical Branch; and Anna Wilson, professor of pediatrics at the Oregon Health & Science University.

LIVING WITH RHEUMATOID ARTHRITIS

Deb Constien, diagnosed with rheumatoid arthritis (RA) at age 13, said pain and fatigue have been part of her life for the past 43 years. Fortunately, the era of biologic medications for RA has been a game changer for her and her 26-year-old son, who also has RA, as these medications have stopped the progression of their disease. Nonetheless, living with RA means thinking through and prioritizing daily activities and allocating tasks to others to accommodate the energy-limiting nature of the disease. "You have to think and prioritize every movement you make," she said.

Constien said she is a volunteer with the Outcome Measures in Rheumatology (OMERACT) group, a global, volunteer-driven, not-for-profit organization committed to improving outcomes for patients with autoimmune and musculoskeletal diseases through advancing the design and quality of clinical studies.[1] This group has collaborated with patients to identify three important domains for clinical trials: pain, fatigue, and independence.

One challenge, said Constien, is that each person with RA has a different experience dealing with limitations in physical function and participating in life. RA patients struggle with having control over their lives and with needing assistance, she said, because assistance can be both supportive and independence-limiting. Constien also mentioned how the role of shame associated with having a disability interfered with utilizing necessary support services and accommodations, such as Social Security Disability Insurance. For example, Constien emphasized hesitancy to use elevators as opposed to stairs and reluctance to use a handicap placard due to the associated stigma of being a person with a disability. Finally, she stressed the importance of involving patients in research and gaining their perspectives, since they are the experts in the experience of living with chronic pain.

CURRENT EVIDENCE TO SUPPORT BEST PRACTICES IN MEASURING AND ASSESSING CHRONIC PAIN

Steven George said there is substantial evidence delinking anatomic pathology from pain severity. As a result, imaging is not recommended for diagnosing non-specific and nociplastic spine-related pain and making treatment decisions. He noted that because evidence linking anatomy with pain is weak, there is limited value in using diagnostic terms such as "discogenic," "facet joint," "sacroiliac," or even "osteoarthritis" for pain assessment. Rather than being driven by anatomy, the pain sensation has several contributors, including modulation by the nervous system; contextual factors such as pain beliefs, expectations, and the placebo effect; cognitive factors including attention, distraction, hypervigilance, and catastrophizing; and mood (Figure 4-1).

George said substantial evidence supports the nervous system's influence on developing and maintaining chronic pain, suggesting chronic pain is a nervous system disease (George and Bishop, 2018). As a result, there is a great deal of interest in quantifying nervous system processing of nociception using quantitative sensory testing. This type of testing, he explained, is a form of psychophysical testing that assesses somatosensory function by measuring how individuals respond to controlled, standardized stimuli (MacKichan et al., 2008). This move toward assessment of nervous system processing, said George, is consistent with the evidence. However, there is likely limited value in assessing pain related to disability because

---

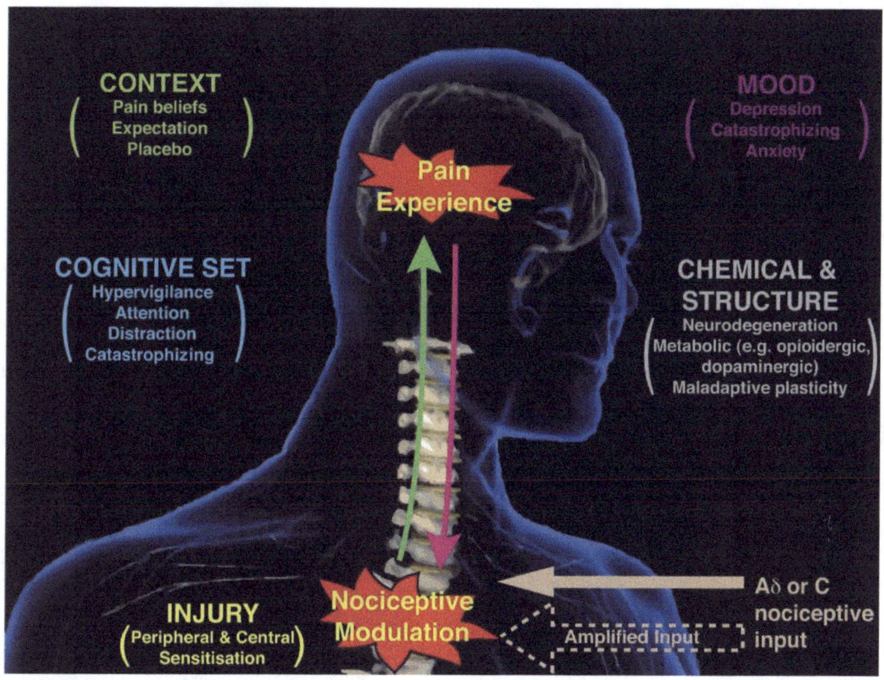

FIGURE 4-1 The multiple factors contributing to pain.
SOURCES: George presentation, April 17, 2025; Tracey and Mantyh, 2007, used with permission from Elsevier.

such an assessment is good at measuring the response to a painful stimulus but not as good at measuring the pain itself.

Pain-related disability assessment, said George, needs to be more than measuring the ability to feel pain. Rather, it needs to measure the interference or impact pain has on an individual's life. Pain measurement that considers interference or impact has two key components: the number of days of pain an individual experiences in a set period and how frequently pain interferes with activities. One example of a graded chronic pain scale uses the number of days in the past three months as the primary differentiator, along with responses from the Pain, Enjoyment of Life, and General Activity Scale (Von Korff et al., 2020). These measurements allow standardization, which in turn enables comparison across different populations and conditions. The data from these measurements may have important implications for disability assessment.

George ended his presentation with a caveat: The science supporting the use of physical performance measures, such as Functional Capacity

Evaluations, to determine how much pain is affecting performance, and thus disability or functional levels, is dubious. Evidence does support using self-report measures for assessing pain, and measures that assess pain impact and interference may be relevant for disability determination.

PREVALENCE AND IMPACT OF CHRONIC PAIN IN CHILDHOOD

In 2024, said Anna Wilson, a systematic review of data from 119 studies representing more than 1 million children found that 20 percent of children and adolescents experienced chronic pain lasting three months or longer, with the highest prevalence for headaches and musculoskeletal pain (Chambers et al., 2024). She added that some 5 to 8 percent of children experience moderate to severe functional impairment in activity, engagement, peer relationships, and school attendance resulting from pain, with the prevalence increasing with age and peaking at 14 to 15 years old. Wilson noted that U.S. health care expenditures associated with pediatric pain-related conditions total in the billions, with decade-old estimates ranging from $12 billion (Groenewald et al., 2015) to $20 billion (Groenewald et al., 2014), about double the cost of asthma.

Wilson said sex differences begin around puberty and persist into adulthood, with females reporting more high-impact chronic pain than males. Adults with chronic pain often report onset during childhood, and follow-up assessment of adolescents with chronic pain has shown that pain problems persist into adulthood. The highest rates of persistence occur among children who experience high pain frequency and interference. Moreover, adults with childhood pain onset have higher pain-related disability compared to those with adult onset. She emphasized, however, that just because pain persists across the lifespan does not mean there is no lifespan variability in individual patients over time.

Wilson noted the results of one study that assembled children with chronic pain, their parents, and medical providers to reach consensus about the outcome measures needed for clinical trials of pain interventions in children (Palermo et al., 2021). By unanimous vote, the assembled group recommended that pain severity, pain interference with daily living, overall well-being, and adverse events should be mandatory domains that all trials assess. "Starting with these core domains is a great place not just for clinical trials but for any comprehensive assessment of children's pain," said Wilson.

She noted that children's pain occurs in the context of their parents and family, as well as the broader social and cultural contexts. Thus, assessment needs to consider these factors, as well as how pain interferes with typical development and participation in age-appropriate social roles and activities. Wilson and her colleagues have identified an intergenerational risk for pain, with children with pain being highly likely to have at least one parent with chronic pain (Higgins et al., 2015). In addition, off-spring of parents with chronic pain have higher pain levels. Both genetics and shared environments seem to play a role here.

In an ongoing study, Wilson and her collaborators are looking at the effect of maternal chronic pain on children (Stone et al., 2019). What the data have shown so far is that chronic pain affects the physical aspects of parenting, the mother's involvement in the child's activities, and the mother's emotions related to parenting. She noted that childhood is an opportunity to prevent chronic pain in adulthood, as well as to provide patients with coping mechanisms and ways of managing pain that can help them across the lifespan.

IMPLICATIONS FOR SOCIAL SECURITY DISABILITY DETERMINATIONS

Carole Tucker said children as young as eight years old are reliable and consistent reporters of their health conditions using self-report measures such as face pain scales, the pediatric pain questionnaire, Bath Adolescent Pain Questionnaire, and Pain Catastrophizing Scale for children. However, it is important to take a multidimensional approach to pain assessment because children's expression of pain differs significantly across developmental stages. This makes standardized assessment challenging for Social Security Administration (SSA) determinations.

Tucker said pain in children has neurophysiological effects on their development, including physically altered movement patterns, psychological anxiety, depression, and strained social and peer relationships. While developing social and peer relationships is a key hallmark of healthy, functioning children, the electronic health record (EHR) does not accurately reflect those relationships. Thus, making a disability determination based primarily on medical diagnoses in the EHR serves children poorly.

Multidisciplinary measurement involves assessing different domains as well as getting those assessments from a variety of professionals, including medical specialists, physical and occupational therapists, psychologists, school personnel, and social workers. Getting important information from the school environment, however, is "a nightmare," said Tucker, because states regulate who can collect and use school-generated data.

Tucker said several types of clinical outcome assessments could be useful for disability determinations (Figure 4-2). In her opinion, outcome assessments based on patient-reported outcomes should be weighed more heavily than those based on observational reports. At the same time, performance outcomes are helpful because they assess the impact of pain on function and participation.

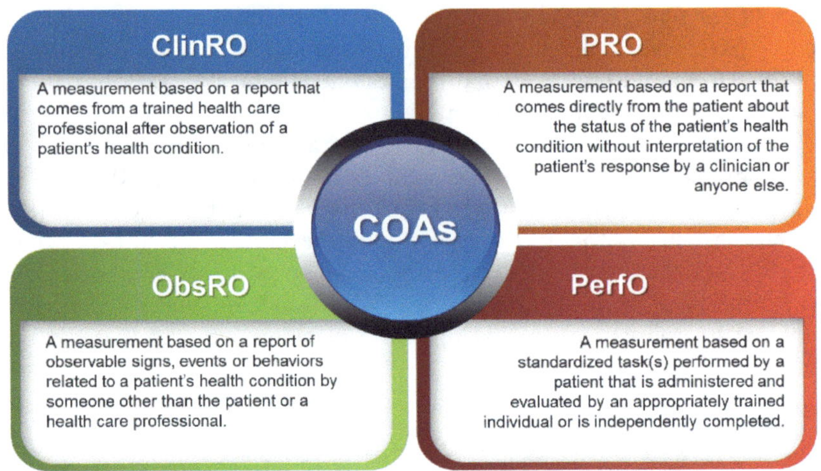

FIGURE 4-2 Types of clinical outcome assessments (COAs).
SOURCE: Tucker presentation, April 17, 2025; FDA, 2018.

If pressed to recommend gold-standard measures for assessing pain in children, Tucker said such measures would need to be developmentally appropriate, account for the child's developmental stages, and include information from the child, parents, clinician, schools, and others involved with the child. The measures would be multidimensional, assessing pain intensity, location, quality, frequency, duration, and functional impact, and include context-specific measures appropriate for different settings. Finally, they would be longitudinal and include regular assessment over time rather than at a single point. "For Social Security disability determinations, the combination of standardized self-report measures, functional assessment tools, and school and home functioning documentation provide the most comprehensive evidence base," said Tucker.

After noting challenges with the current SSA framework for pediatric chronic pain, Tucker recommended several improvements SSA could make. These included using enhanced assessment protocols, relying on cross-system collaboration, improving transition planning from childhood to adult, and issuing guidance updates. "Children with chronic pain face unique assessment challenges that impact their access to appropriate disability determinations," she said. "By improving our measurement tools, documentation systems, and cross-disciplinary collaboration, we can better serve this vulnerable population and ensure appropriate support through the Social Security disability system."

5

Considering Best Practices and Clinician Perspectives on Chronic Pain Treatment and Management in Children

In this session participants discussed best practices and methods of categorizing chronic pain and advancements in the treatment, management, and measurement of children's chronic pain levels. They also highlighted special considerations in how medical providers approach treatment of different severities in chronic pain in children. The speakers were Casey Cashman, director of the Pediatric Pain Warriors Program at U.S. Pain Foundation; Tonya Palermo, professor and vice chair for research, anesthesiology, and pain medicine at the University of Washington; Stefan Friedrichsdorf, medical director of the Stad Center for Pediatric Pain, Palliative and Integrative Medicine at Benioff Children's Hospitals in Oakland and San Francisco; and Laura Simons, professor of anesthesiology, perioperative, and pain medicine at Stanford University Medical School.

LIVING WITH MULTIPLE SERIOUS HEALTH CONDITIONS, INCLUDING COMPLEX REGIONAL PAIN SYNDROME

Casey Cashman, who said she does not remember a time when she was not dealing with strange medical issues, said having a family who believed in her and a pediatrician who did not dismiss what she was going through made all the difference. Today, while she deals with several serious health conditions, including complex regional pain syndrome, people tell her she does not look like she is in pain. The truth is that pain is invisible, and just because someone is smiling does not mean they are not struggling, Cashman said. She has been fortunate to have access to experimental treatments, such as hyperbaric oxygen therapy and ketamine infusions, but

21

these are expensive, rare, and not available to everyone, so many people go without.

Cashman stressed how important it is to believe what children are saying about their pain, to support them and their families, and to not make them fight for the care they need. "We need to change the way our health care system sees pain, especially in young people, because if we can change the pain journey for children, we can change their whole life," she said. Having accepted that she will never be pain free, she has hope that life is manageable and that she can have a life with joy, purpose, and love.

PSYCHOLOGICAL INTERVENTIONS FOR YOUTH WITH CHRONIC PAIN

Tonya Palermo listed the four transformative goals of the Lancet Child and Adolescent Health Commission, developed for the field of pediatric pain:

- Make pain matter by improving equity, eliminating stigma, and making pain matter to everyone, including health professionals, policy makers, funders, researchers, clinicians, and society at large.
- Make pain understood by improving knowledge of all types of pain across the life course and integrating biological, psychological, and social elements.
- Make pain visible by standardizing assessments for pain and determining pain status in every child.
- Make pain better by avoiding unnecessary pain, preventing the transition from acute to chronic pain, and striving for universal access to effective pain treatments for children and adolescents.

Palermo said there are beliefs and biases about childhood pain that reinforce stigma and delay treatment, particularly the tendency to disbelieve children and adolescents about their pain experience that can make the journey to find pain care more challenging (Wakefield et al., 2022). She noted how important it is to recognize the potential long-term effects of adolescent chronic pain on adult educational, vocational, and social outcomes. Additional research has shown that someone with chronic pain during adolescence is less likely to receive a high school diploma, bachelor's degree, and employer-provided insurance benefits, and more likely to receive public assistance or disability payments, become pregnant or a parent earlier, and have lower relationship satisfaction as young adults (Murray et al., 2020).

A wide range of neurobiological, emotional, social, family, and health behavior vulnerabilities influence childhood chronic pain. Palermo said these factors predict pain during childhood but also chronic pain maintenance into adulthood, with longitudinal studies showing that 30 to 70 percent of children with pain continue to experience it into adulthood. Therefore, prevention and management of chronic pain must begin in childhood, Palermo said, and her focus as a psychologist has been on identifying and targeting vulnerabilities that psychological treatment approaches can address (Palermo, 2020). She explained that, compared to those without pain, children and adolescents with chronic pain have three times the increased risk of developing mental health conditions, including anxiety and depressive disorders, posttraumatic stress disorder, suicidality, and substance use disorder.

Fortunately, said Palermo, robust evidence supports the use of psychological therapies to manage chronic pain in childhood, most of which are based on cognitive behavioral therapy (CBT; Fisher et al., 2018). CBT-based therapies teach children and families skills for self-managing and coping with pain and focus on enhancing functioning in daily life, including supporting re-engagement in school, social life, and physical activity. Unfortunately, only 5 percent of children and adolescents with chronic pain will receive a psychological intervention, largely because of a shortage of interdisciplinary pediatric pain clinics and pain psychologists, delayed referral to subspecialty care, and long waiting lists for pain services.

To address the availability problem, Palermo developed and tested an internet-delivered, family-based CBT program, WebMAP, for reducing adolescent pain-related disability and depression and anxiety symptoms (Palermo et al., 2009; Walker et al., 2021). This program improved parents' perceptions of the effects of chronic pain and helped change parental protective behaviors. Specialty clinics have implemented a mobile app version of WebMAP and achieved high adoption and sustainability (Palermo et al., 2020). The free app, also available in a Spanish version, is available in both Apple and Google app stores.

While schools would be an ideal setting for implementing this type of intervention, Palermo said the lack of standardized guidelines and resources for school personnel to effectively support students with chronic pain is a major impediment. Researchers have conducted few school-based interventions, but Palermo said there are opportunities to embed pain education and intervention in existing school-based mental health programs, such as mindfulness courses and adverse childhood experience training.

Palermo noted the need to make low-cost, low-intensity interventions universally available to help children with chronic pain in multiple settings of care. "Early intervention and prevention are really key to having a population-level impact on pain," she said.

PREVALENCE OF CHRONIC PAIN IN CHILDREN

Stefan Friedrichsdorf said 3 to 5 percent—444,000 to 740,000—of U.S. children and adolescents develop significant pain-related disability and need intensive pain rehabilitation (Huguet and Miró, 2008). Between 12 and 20 percent of pediatric inpatients show features of chronic pain (Friedrichsdorf et al., 2015; Postier et al., 2018), he added. Primary chronic pain disorders in children include chronic migraines and tension-type headaches, chronic abdominal pain, and widespread chronic musculoskeletal pain.

Friedrichsdorf said surgery is usually not recommended to address chronic pain in children and adolescents. In fact, there are data showing that adolescents who had surgery for lumbar disk herniation experienced worse pain and other health complications in adulthood (Lagerbäck et al., 2021; Ruehr et al., 2024). He noted that children in pain develop more stress and anxiety, which causes a vicious cycle of more pain, triggering more stress and anxiety and more pain. Eventually, these children develop avoidance behaviors that make them less active, then lose conditioning and develop a faster heart rate when they are active.

An important factor in treating children with chronic pain, said Friedrichsdorf, is that these children hear their pain is real, as young people often experience pain for over 2 years before getting a diagnosis (Neville et al., 2020).

Friedrichsdorf explained that a rehabilitative pediatric pain clinic approach includes physical therapy, integrative medicine techniques, psychotherapy, family coaching, and normalizing life activities such as sleeping, having fun, and attending school full time. There is little emphasis on pharmacotherapy, particularly using opioids. This cost-effective approach enables many children treated in pediatric outpatient pain clinics to return to everyday function, with some needing additional intensive treatment such as additional rehabilitative day treatment or an inpatient program (Evans et al., 2016; Friedrichsdorf et al., 2016; Mahrer et al., 2018; Simons et al., 2018). However, there are fewer than ten pediatric programs in the United States that offer this approach. In fact, there are only 60 self-declared pediatric pain clinics in 32 states and the District of Columbia (Figure 5-1).

CONSIDERING INNOVATIVE APPROACHES FOR THE TREATMENT OF CHRONIC PAIN IN CHILDREN

Laura Simons said one way to treat young people more efficiently, given the shortage of pediatric pain specialists and pain clinics, is to use brief screening tools to triage risk level (Simons et al., 2015; Heathcote et al., 2018). This allows children to get into appropriate treatment pro-

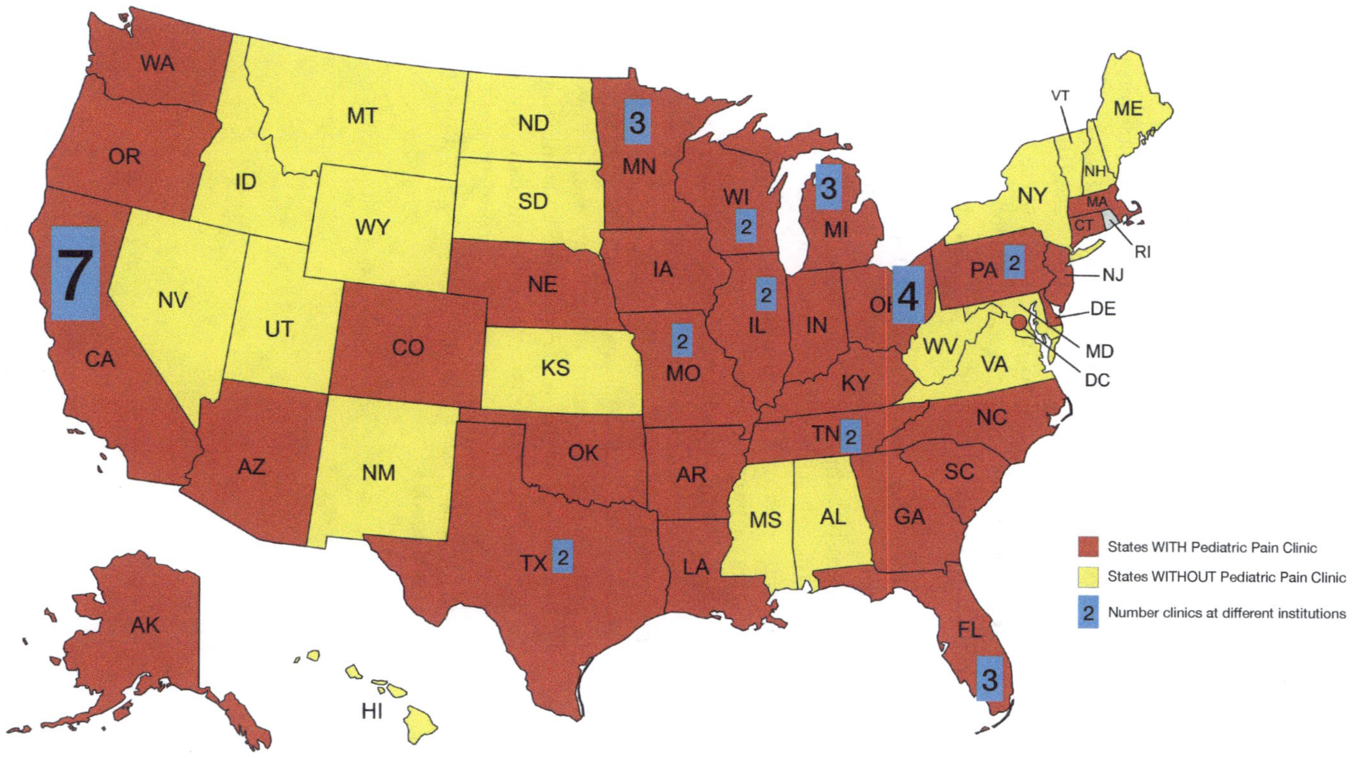

FIGURE 5-1 U.S. pediatric pain clinics, 2025.
SOURCE: Friedrichsdorf presentation, April 17, 2025. Based on data from Palermo, T. "International Directory of Pediatric Chronic Pain Programs." Published December 23, 2024 at http://childpain.org/index.php/resources.

grams. One program she has been using is the two-hour virtual Empowered Relief®[1] class adapted for youth, which helps validate the pain these children are experiencing, teaches them about how the brain processes pain, provides them with simple daily skills, and helps them create a personalized plan for long-term relief.

The Empowered Relief® program adapted for youth prepares children who need more intensive interventions. One intervention she has been working on is Graded Exposure Treatment (GET) Living, which integrates pain psychology and physical therapy to help young people regain their functionality (Simons et al., 2020). This intervention has also been modified to deliver GET Living digitally and to incorporate virtual reality into pain rehabilitation as a means of increasing engagement in what can be a boring, uncomfortable, and painful experience (Griffin et al., 2020; Simons et al., 2024).

As Friedrichsdorf noted, some patients will need more intensive rehabilitation programs. However, said Simons, even with more intensive programs, her data show that between one-third and half of young people continue to experience chronic pain, though with improved functionality (Simons et al., 2013, 2018). The challenge is emphasizing different aspects of an intensive interdisciplinary approach to pain treatment depending on an individual's particular need (Figure 5-2). "I think there is so much promise in our ability to use predictive analytics and patient-centered precision care to have a better understanding of who needs what," she said.

Simons said a young person's journey with chronic pain is long and complex. It is critical, she said, that young people can access low-burden, scalable behavioral health interventions, and that current innovative approaches to screening and comprehensive assessment can inform individualized treatment approaches. A meaningful subgroup of patients will require intensive interdisciplinary pain treatment, which is of limited availability today, she acknowledged.

---

[1] https://empoweredrelief.stanford.edu/ (accessed June 19, 2025).

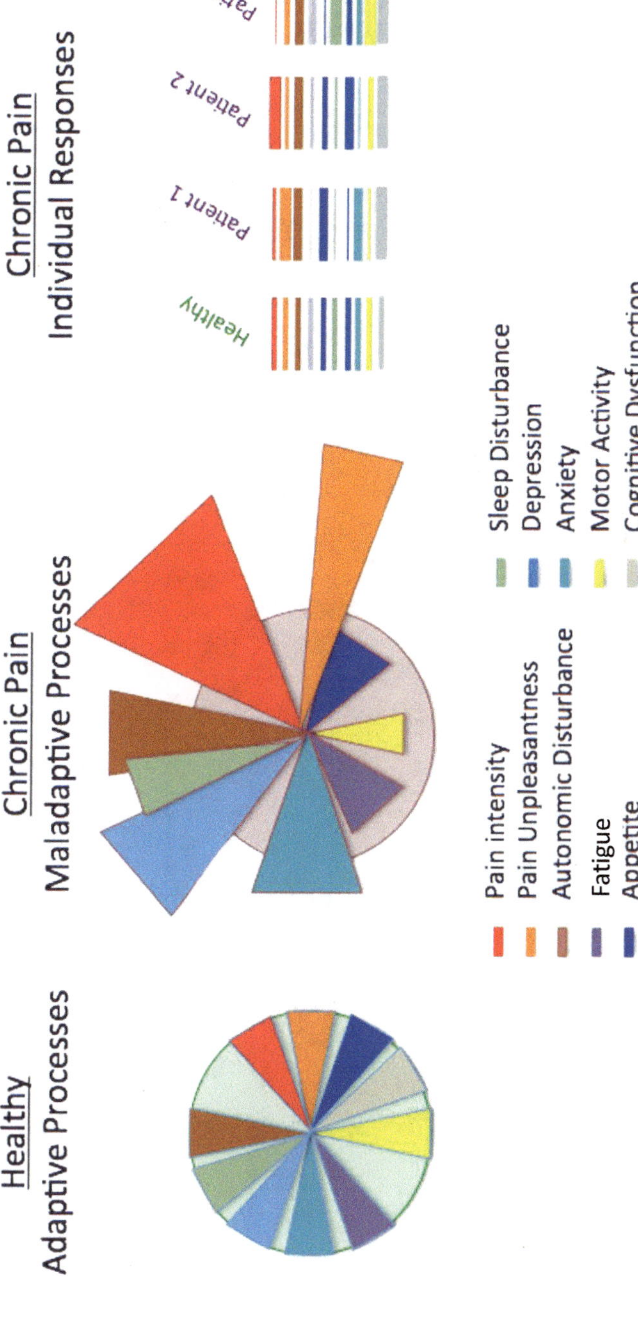

FIGURE 5-2 Applying an individual lens for patient-centered pain care.
SOURCES: Simons presentation, April 17, 2025. Adapted from Borsook and Kalso, 2013.

6

Considering Best Practices on Chronic Pain Treatment and Management in Adults

The workshop's fourth session discussed best practices and methods of categorizing chronic pain; advances in treating, managing, and measuring adults' pain levels; and how much various types of chronic pain treatments alleviate functional limitations. The speakers were Kemly Philip, division chief of musculoskeletal and interventional pain and assistant professor, Department of Physical Medicine and Rehabilitation at the UTHealth McGovern Medical School; Carol Greco, associate professor of psychiatry and physical therapy at the University of Pittsburgh; and Julie Fritz, distinguished professor of physical therapy and athletic training at the University of Utah.

AN OVERVIEW OF CHRONIC PAIN IN ADULTS

After reviewing what previous speakers had discussed about the nature of chronic pain and its effects on decreasing function and increasing disability, Kemly Philip explained that acute and chronic pain management should be individualized, multimodal, and multidisciplinary (Pain Management Best Practices Inter-Agency Task Force, 2019). Management should include a combination of medication, restorative therapies, interventional procedures, behavioral health approaches, and complementary and integrative health approaches.

The most recent guidelines from the Centers for Disease Control and Prevention recommend starting with non-opioids such as nonsteroidal anti-inflammatories or anti-convulsants as first-line therapies for adults with chronic pain and to use the lowest effective dose of these analgesics

29

(McDonagh et al., 2020). If opioids are needed, it is imperative to ensure the benefits outweigh the risks, said Philip, by using risk assessment tools and an opioid pain medication agreement.

She noted there is a large variety of image-guided interventions that can be used to both identify and treat sources of pain. Such interventions include joint and peripheral nerve injections, epidural steroid injections, radiofrequency ablation, neuromodulation, and others. These interventions have fewer systemic side effects compared to pharmacologic interventions; they limit the need for pharmacologic interventions or surgery (U.S. Department of Health and Human Services, 2019); and when combined with therapy, they produce a synergistic benefit (Kraal et al., 2018). Philip said that between 2000 and 2013, use of interventional pain procedures increased by 236 percent among fee-for-service Medicare beneficiaries (Manchikanti et al., 2015).

CHRONIC PAIN MANAGEMENT FROM A PSYCHOLOGIST'S PERSPECTIVE

Carol Greco discussed the biopsychosocial model of pain and its importance for understanding an individual's pain experience and needs. The biopsychosocial model of pain holds that pain is complex and that many biological, psychological, and social factors influence it. She explained that pain is experienced in a personal, psychological, and social context, and understanding an individual patient's context can help better tailor a treatment plan and lead to better outcomes. The medical setting and system, the clinic personnel, and the clinical provider are all part of the social context of pain and its treatment.

Greco listed several approaches to assessing an individual's beliefs about pain, including the Fear Avoidance Belief Questionnaire, the Pain Catastrophizing Scale to identify unhelpful beliefs about pain, the Chronic Pain Acceptance Questionnaire to assess resilience, and the STarT Back Screening Tool for low back pain.

There is a good evidence base, said Greco, to support the use of psychological approaches for treating chronic pain and illness symptoms. These include cognitive behavioral therapy (CBT; Gatchel and Rollings, 2008), acceptance and commitment therapy (ACT; McCracken and Vowles, 2014; Ma et al., 2023), and mindfulness-based stress reduction (MBSR; Qaseem et al., 2017; Skelly et al., 2020). CBT, said Greco, aligns with the biopsychosocial model, is patient-centered, and requires the patient to be an active participant in treatment. It addresses the cognitive, emotional, and behavioral dimensions of chronic pain by helping the patient reconceptualize the pain. CBT targets unhelpful thought patterns, such as "I will never get better," through cognitive reframing and building new habits and brain pathways. ACT, a variation of CBT, is driven more by the patient's self-defined values and what is hindering moving toward those. ACT is based on acceptance and mindfulness and being willing to engage in activities even though pain is present.

MBSR, a favorite of Greco's, is an eight-week, group-based psycho-education program that uses secular meditation methods to reduce reactivity to pain and stress and increase coping ability. MBSR also includes home practice, using mindfulness in one's daily life, and stretching. The American College of Physicians and Agency for Healthcare Research and Quality both recommend MBSR for chronic low back pain. Greco cited several studies showing that adults participating in MBSR experienced more improvement in pain symptoms compared to control groups (Morone et al., 2009; Greco et al., 2021).

Greco has also been involved in research integrating psychosocial methods into physical therapy treatment and training physical therapists and chiropractors to add biopsychosocial self-management methods into their practices. These include patient-centered communication, shared decision making, and relaxation strategies (Farrokhi et al., 2020; Delitto et al., 2021; Main et al., 2023; Leininger et al., 2025).

Greco said that psychological treatments should not replace other treatments. It is important, she added, to understand the billing limits within the health care system for psychological treatments for chronic pain. One potential problem is that psychologists, social workers, and counselors use mental health diagnostic and billing codes, which could lead to the assumption that the patient has a mental health problem, not a physical health condition.

CLINICIAN PERSPECTIVES ON CHRONIC PAIN TREATMENT AND MANAGEMENT IN ADULTS

Julie Fritz identified the various ways adults manage chronic pain based on data from a national survey (Figure 6-1; Rikard et al., 2023). What stood out to her from these data was that a primary intervention involved unsupervised exercise. She noted that a recent systematic review of 301 studies on 56 treatments for low back pain found that only about 10 percent of the treatments had a measurable benefit on pain intensity, though exercise was effective.

Fritz said the finding that exercise had a positive benefit of modest magnitude is consistent across chronic pain conditions (Skelly et al., 2020; Hayden et al., 2021). The challenge is identifying the right type and amount of exercise for a specific type of chronic pain and determining how to combine that with a psychological intervention. What does matter for effectiveness is adherence to whatever exercise or behavioral regimen is prescribed (Jones et al., 2025).

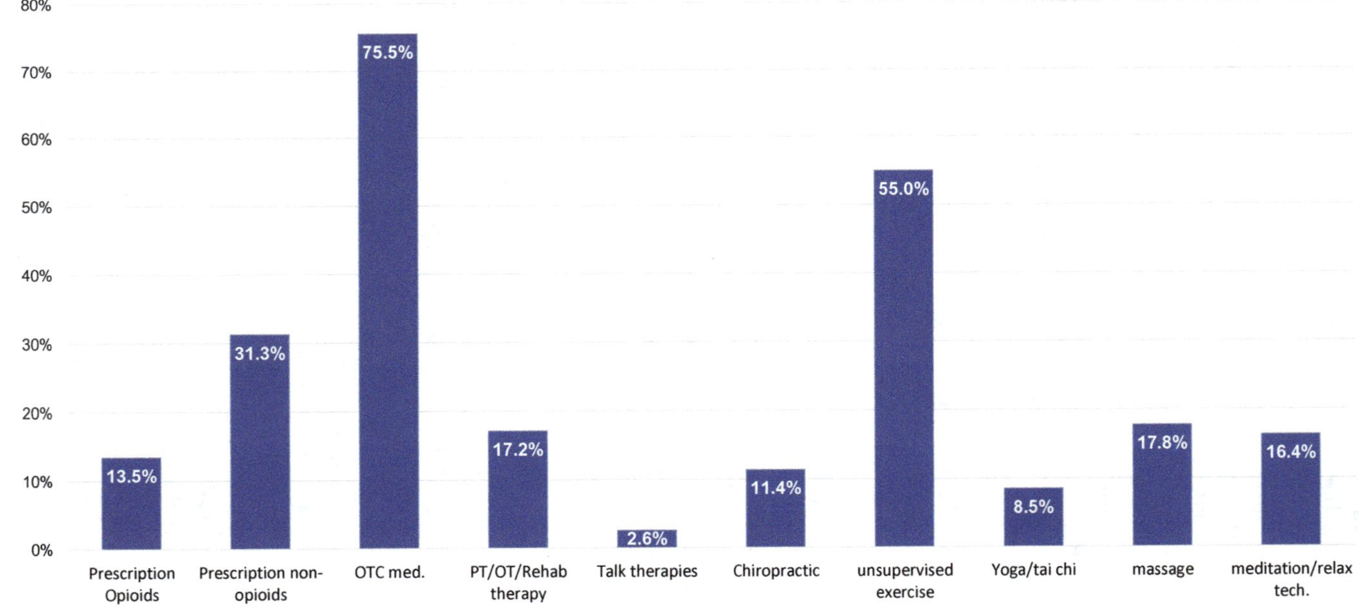

FIGURE 6-1 Prevalence of pain management therapy use during the past three months among adults with chronic pain, 2020.
SOURCES: Fritz presentation, April 17, 2025; Data from Rikard et al., 2023.

There are other considerations regarding what makes exercise more effective (Alaiti et al., 2022; Wood et al., 2024). Despite purported differences in mechanisms, said Fritz, many exercise interventions across different pain conditions share mediators such as self-efficacy, fear of movement, and pain beliefs. Adherence and outcomes of exercise likely improve when the mechanisms of trust, motivation, and confidence are used to enhance therapeutic alliance. In addition, exercise prescribed in a way that is tailored to an individual's goals, with personalized advice, education, and reassurance, can increase motivation and adherence.

Fritz said the specific exercise may not matter as much as developing a personalized plan to which the person can adhere. Supervised exercise programs, such as those with a physical therapist, can be particularly beneficial when provided as part of a tailored multimodal intervention in a manner that builds a therapeutic alliance and intrinsic motivation for behavior change. The optimal therapeutic alliance, she explained, is achieved when both the patient and provider agree on the goals of treatment and the methods to achieve positive health outcomes (Ardito and Rabellino, 2011).

7

Patient Journeys and Clinician Perspectives in Treating and Managing Chronic Pain

In the fifth session participants discussed the lived experiences of people with chronic pain as they navigate the Social Security Administration disability system. The session also highlighted special considerations for how medical providers approach treatment of chronic pain of different severities in adults. The speakers were Anna Williams, vice president, Clusterbusters; Joseph Cammilleri, clinical specialist in ambulatory care pain management at University of Florida Health Jacksonville; and Shravani Durbhakula, comprehensive pain service medical director, Vanderbilt University School of Medicine.

THE LIVED EXPERIENCE OF CHRONIC PAIN

Anna Williams grew up on a farm in rural West Virginia. Her family did not have health insurance, and although she experienced abdominal pain, headaches, and persistent chronic pain during her menstrual cycle, the first time she saw a doctor for chronic pain was at age 19, when she was in college. She was diagnosed then with fibromyalgia and migraine, and thanks to insurance, she was able to start treatment. However, at age 23, her symptoms worsened, and even walking became difficult, causing her to lose her job and insurance. The community health clinicians she saw dismissed her symptoms as an "it-is-all-in-your-head kind of thing." She felt unheard and humiliated.

After spending over two years going through the process of enrolling under the Social Security Disability Insurance program, she was granted eligibility. This enabled her to see a doctor and resume proper treatment.

35

In the years since, she married, and thanks to her husband's health insurance, she was able to maintain continuity of care; but following surgery for bilateral torn hip labrums, she began experiencing cluster headaches. During that time, she was once again denied disability coverage—one letter said she was denied because she could be a dishwasher. "To me, that was just heartless, and it made things difficult for me," said Williams.

At age 42, Williams was diagnosed with bilateral trigeminal neuralgia, which feels like she has a drill boring into her jaw, a sensation that can last for hours to weeks. Because she has struggled to find care locally, telehealth has been a huge help for her, even though she must pay for it herself. "They listen, they believe me, and they think outside the box for treatments," said Williams.

TREATING CHRONIC PAIN IN UNINSURED PATIENTS: A PHARMACIST'S PERSPECTIVE

Joseph Cammilleri said there are few options for treating an uninsured individual who suffers from chronic pain. "We are limited to medication management for our [uninsured] patients, and while sometimes we can get them into physical therapy, it is just going to be for maybe two or three visits," said Cammilleri. Motivational interviewing and medication management become the focus for these individuals, he added.

Cammilleri, who received training as a pain pharmacist, said he sees chronic pain patients after they receive a pain diagnosis from their primary care physician. He can spend 30 to 60 minutes with a patient, providing time for the in-depth education many of these individuals need. "And when we are talking about medication therapy management, we are the medication experts," he said.

One of the biggest challenges for pharmacological pain management is that there are no clear guidelines other than starting with nonpharmacologic and non-opioid therapy, said Cammilleri. "There is nothing that says one medication will work better than another, and the data show minimal effects for pretty much all medication," he noted. In his opinion, the subjective nature of pain scores and individual response to a given pain medication are part of the problem that leads to trial-and-error approaches. Primary care physicians, he said, have limited time to do a complete pain assessment, even as they must oversee more chronic pain cases given the shortage of pain physicians.

Even for patients with insurance, finding a pain specialist who will take in-network insurance is an obstacle, as is getting them approved for nonpharmacologic options such as cognitive behavioral therapy or pain coaching. Inadequate care transitions can be another barrier when a patient needs to switch physicians, and medication access can be a major impediment. Analgesic shortages, insurance formularies, prior authorizations, cost, and the stigma associated with opioids can be significant barriers to pain management.

Given these obstacles and the struggle individuals with chronic pain experience to receive appropriate care, it is not surprising that patients become disengaged and lose hope. Establishing trust with a new patient is key, said Cammilleri, and trust starts with believing the patient. Trust also needs to be bidirectional, and when it comes to opioid medication, it is key to trust but verify, he said. He lays out expectations, conducts urine drug screens, counts medication, and frames an individual's treatment plan options based on safety.

IMPROVING ACCESS TO PAIN CARE: A PUBLIC HEALTH OPPORTUNITY

Shravani Durbhakula said new chronic pain cases are outpacing new cases of diabetes, depression, and hypertension (Nahin et al., 2023), yet only 46.9 percent of chronic pain patients receive regular care, compared to 78.8 percent of diabetics (National Center for Health Statistics, 2023). In 2023 there were 5,871 pain medicine physicians in the United States, which means there were nearly 56,500 potential pain patients for each pain physician, compared to fewer than 15,000 potential cardiology patients per cardiologist and just over 20,000 cancer patients per oncologist (Durbhakula et al., 2024). As a result, there is an average 7.8-year delay to receive pain specialty care, during which time a patient might see eight other clinicians. Some 20 percent of those with chronic pain never reach a pain specialist (Rufener et al., 2024).

Rural areas, said Durbhakula, have a higher pain prevalence but less access to pain specialists. This means that most pain care is delivered by primary care physicians and other health care professionals who lack formal pain training. In Tennessee, where she practices, many pain clinics were shuttered because of questionable opioid dispensing practices, which means that those patients were most likely not receiving appropriate care in the first place and now have even less access to proper care.

One of Durbhakula's patients, a woman in her 80s, was in a complete 10-year remission from cancer but was still on high-dose opioid therapy because she had shoulder pain. She came to Durbhakula because nobody else would renew her opioid prescription, but neither had anyone tried to wean her from opioids even though she wanted to do so. Durbhakula assisted her through the process and designed other forms of treatment that gave her excellent pain relief.

One issue is that there are system gaps in pain education, starting with a lack of prioritization, said Durbhakula. The average U.S. medical student receives 11 hours of pain education, and only 4 percent of U.S. medical schools are offering a dedicated pain course (Mezei and Murinson, 2011). There are no shared standards for pain education, and there has been a 45 percent decline in pain fellowship applications since 2019, with only 67.6 percent of pain fellowship programs filled in 2024 (Pritzlaff et al., 2025). In contrast, when she was training over a decade ago, pain medicine was the most competitive specialty in anesthesiology residency. There have been efforts to improve medical education. For instance, at Johns Hopkins School of Medicine, Durbhakula directed a mandatory 20-hour pain course for all first-year students, which shifted the students' attitudes toward pain patients and reduced the stigma of treating pain (Durbhakula et al., 2024). However, Durbhakula noted, these efforts to increase education of pain management are not standardized, comprehensive, or widespread, nor are there education curricula related to pain management and disability determinations for medical school students to further understand the connections between chronic pain and the disability system.

Durbhakula said the lack of access to pain specialists, lack of pain education for primary care clinicians, stigma associated with treating pain patients, and insufficient insurance coverage for alternative treatment approaches have led to inadequate pain care and increased suffering. These have also led to avoidable disability, creating public health and economic issues. Addressing this public health problem will require a systems-level approach going forward, said Durbhakula. It is imperative to expand primary care physician training on pain management, standardize medical school pain education—including education on disability determinations in U.S. medical schools—incentivize pain employment in rural areas, ensure evidence-based insurance coverage and denials, and increase access to telehealth and virtual care, noted Durbhakula. Finally, there is a need for remote management platforms and digital self-management tools with assistance from artificial intelligence (Piette et al., 2022).

8

Health Care System Challenges in Comprehensive Chronic Pain Management

The first session of the workshop's second day covered how the many experiences and challenges related to chronic pain and its management affect health status, functional limitations, and medical records for adults and children. Its discussions also explored systemic barriers to delivering comprehensive, evidence-based pain care across various health care practices. The speakers were Andrea Anderson, patient advocate and advisor to the National Pain Advocacy Center; Beth Darnall, professor of anesthesiology, perioperative, and pain medicine and director of the Stanford Pain Relief Innovations Lab at Stanford University Medical School; Julie Fritz, distinguished professor of physical therapy and athletic training at the University of Utah; and V. G. Vinod Vydiswaran, associate professor of learning health sciences and associate professor of information at the University of Michigan.

PATIENT EXPERIENCES WITH SOCIAL SECURITY DISABILITY

Andrea Anderson became a chronic pain sufferer after she received a surgery planned for someone else rather than the small surgery she was scheduled to have on her lower back. She was fortunate, though, to receive excellent pain management in her community from a pain specialist, enabling her to raise her family and maintain her professional and social obligations.

High-impact chronic pain affects 10.6 million people, or 20 percent of the chronic pain population in the United States (Pitcher et al., 2019). High-impact chronic pain results in substantial restrictions in daily activities, such as being able to work, go to school, or complete daily chores, and typically lasts three months or longer (Pitcher et al., 2019). "It is the kind of pain that feels like you cannot spend another day inside your body—the kind that can take your life hostage if you cannot find a way to manage it," said Anderson.

To prepare for her presentation, Anderson crowdsourced information via multiple social media platforms from hundreds of chronic pain patients who receive or would like to receive Social Security disability. Responses to the first question she asked, about barriers to care, included the following:

- Challenges with qualifying and acceptance, with the average application being denied multiple times, and having to hire an attorney to finally be granted needed services. The average wait for an application review is now 14 months, up from 2–4 months, and the average hold time to speak to a person is now 4.5 hours. Every respondent said their calls are often terminated before they reach a human.
- Lack of access to clinicians and specialists, particularly in health care deserts such as rural communities. Patients on disability in these communities often rely on disability van services to get them to appointments, but many of these programs operate only one day a week and not on the day their clinicians are in the office.
- Insufficient provider networks, as many physicians do not take Medicare or Medicaid patients. In addition, some plans limit patients to seeing one provider per day, which can be a problem for a patient that relies on hired transport to get them to their appointments.
- Financial constraints, with disability payments inadequate for current economic realities. This can create housing instability, a significant health stressor.
- Difficult pharmacy access, particularly if mobility is a challenge or during a natural disaster when patients report having trouble accessing their medications.

Taken together, these barriers usually increase disability-related delays in care that can affect disease progression, worsen health and symptoms, impede an individual's personal agency and independence, and strain family relationships.

Anderson then offered recommendations from the patient community to the Social Security Administration (SSA):

- Increase staff and training to improve wait time for applications to acceptance and time spent on phone and in-person visits.

- Increase reimbursement rates to clinicians who treat people with complex conditions and persistent pain.
- Allow patients to see more than one provider on a single day.
- Allow patients to store emergency medications in case of disaster.
- Increase mail-order pharmacy access.
- Increase cost of living adjustments beyond Medicare premium increases.
- Provide more low-cost housing and transportation options.

ACCESSIBLE BEHAVIORAL PAIN CARE

What is common throughout the journey from acute pain to chronic pain and then into the Social Security disability determination process is a need for behavioral treatment to support the individual, address their pain more completely, and mitigate some of the symptoms and stresses that co-occur throughout this journey, said Beth Darnall. "We know that people who receive intensive behavioral pain treatment do better, but these intensive treatments are inaccessible, and most people are left without [them]," she said. She added that briefer treatment can offer people many benefits and can be administered across a variety of settings.

Darnall noted the International Association for the Study of Pain defines pain as both a noxious sensory and emotional experience, highlighting the importance of treating both the physical and psychological aspects of chronic pain. However, poor access to behavioral treatment leads to incomplete treatment and overmedicalization of chronic pain. In addition, the distress people with chronic pain experience amplifies the pain, allows the pain to progress, and leads to greater disability. While federal agencies and nonprofit organizations have called for better integration of behavioral treatment into pain care pathways and research has shown that integration leads to cost savings (Lanoye et al., 2017; Melek et al., 2018), access to and uptake of behavioral treatment is poor.

Behavioral pain treatment, Darnall explained, is delivered one-on-one or in small groups. Often it involves 16 hours or more of treatment time, during which individuals learn what worsens pain and which daily choices and skills offer the most relief, gain skills and resources to help modulate pain, and create action plans (Darnall, 2019). Barriers to behavioral treatment include the significant time commitment, insurance and copay limitations, work and family obligations, proximity to the treatment site, and a lack of trained clinicians (Darnall et al., 2016). The rise of telehealth during the COVID-19 pandemic has helped somewhat with the proximity issue, she added.

There are also health care system barriers, said Darnall. Often, the health care system emphasizes medical approaches and de-emphasizes behavioral approaches. In addition, reimbursement for behavioral treatment is often insufficient to fully incentivize both adoption and delivery of behavioral treatment and deploy the resources to implement behavioral treatment.

To overcome these barriers, Darnall said the solution is to implement brief treatment approaches. While these approaches may not benefit everyone, they would provide all individuals with chronic pain at least a minimal level of care. She noted there are several benefits of brief treatment for chronic pain (Figure 8-1; Darnall, 2025b), and evidence supports the use of six different brief behavioral treatments for addressing chronic pain (Darnall, 2025b).

Of the six interventions supported by evidence, only two have been adopted widely, largely because clinician training systems are needed to support the adoption and sustainability of these interventions. One of the adopted interventions is brief cognitive behavioral therapy (CBT) for veterans in primary care. It comprises six 30-minute sessions that are integrated with an individual's primary care visits. The second intervention is Empowered Relief®, the only applied intervention adopted widely for nonveterans (Darnall et al., 2021; Ziadni et al., 2021). Empowered Relief® consists of a two-hour didactic session during which people learn three pain management skills and complete a personalized plan. Participants receive access to an app they can use to help them follow their plan.

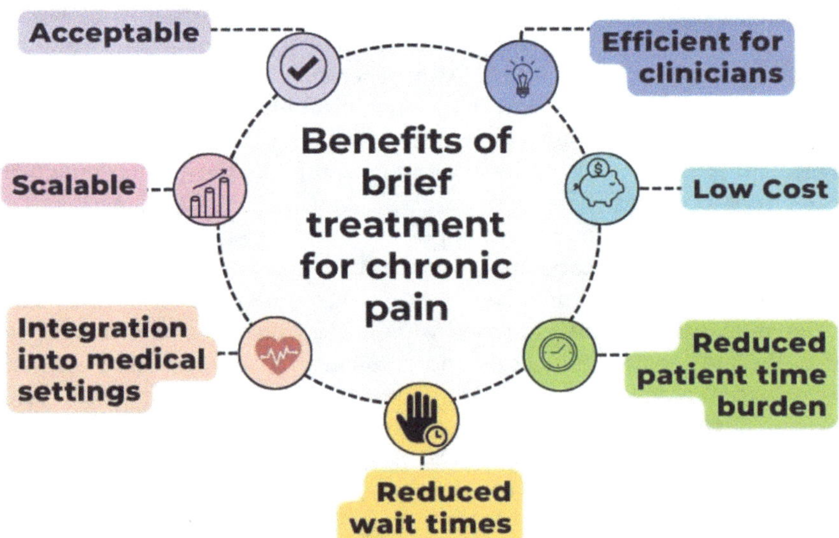

FIGURE 8-1 The benefits of brief treatment for chronic pain.
SOURCE: Darnall presentation, April 18, 2025.

Darnall highlighted the results from several clinical trials comparing this 1-session intervention to an 8-session, 16-hour CBT-based approach, showing that the 1-session intervention produced results equivalent to those produced by the more extensive approach that lasted for at least 6 months (Darnall et al., 2024). There are now some 1,600 certified Empowered Relief® instructors in 30 countries, with 15,000 people visiting the Empowered Relief® app each month. Darnall said most types of licensed clinicians may become certified (Davin et al., 2022; Darnall et al., 2023).

Darnall said providing access to evidence-based behavioral pain treatment is essential, and individuals with chronic pain should receive low-burden behavioral pain treatment early and throughout the Social Security disability determination process. She recommended SSA support research on brief behavioral pain interventions; consider relevant, unsolicited proposals that would relieve pain care gaps; and consider interagency policy advocacy to improve reimbursement across provider types. Finally, she noted that digital interventions integrated into a learning health system could help scale access to behavioral interventions nationally.

HEALTH CARE SYSTEM CHALLENGES IN COMPREHENSIVE CHRONIC PAIN MANAGEMENT

Julie Fritz cited data showing the percentage of adults with chronic pain and high-impact chronic pain increases as the place of residence becomes more rural and family income levels decrease. Federally qualified health centers (FQHCs), which serve medically underserved communities and provide services to all comers on a sliding fee scale, could help meet the demand for chronic pain management services for rural residents and individuals with incomes below the federal poverty line. Fritz noted that in 2023, FQHCs served about 10 percent of the U.S. population (Figure 8-2).

One challenge for FQHCs is a shortage of clinicians trained to provide nonpharmacologic pain treatment for individuals living with chronic pain. FQHCs are attempting to address this shortage using telehealth, particularly in rural settings, though patient access to the necessary technology can be limited. Fritz and her colleagues in Utah have been implementing telehealth for people with chronic pain in the state's rural and underserved urban areas.

She listed several lessons learned in partnering with FQHCs for telehealth pain care (Table 8-1). For example, experience demonstrated the usefulness of incorporating motivational interviewing to produce behavior change and help patients develop coping skills, and to deliver linguistically and ethnically competent care to the state's rural communities.

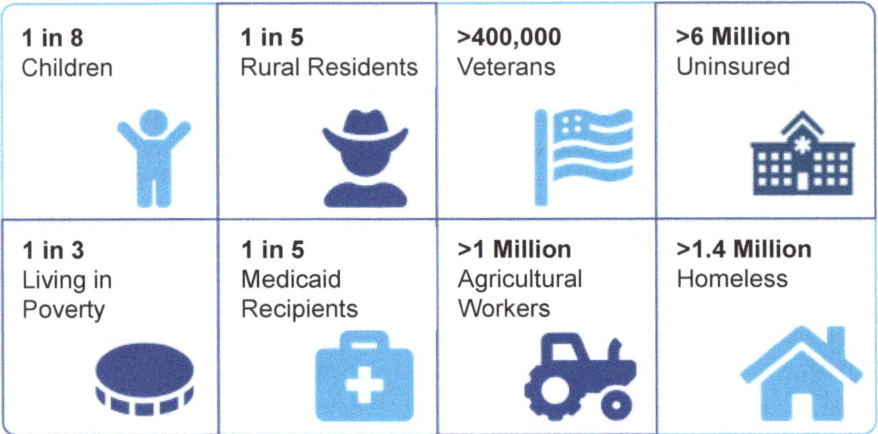

FIGURE 8-2 Demographics of patients served at federally qualified health centers. These centers serve 1 in 10 people in the United States.
SOURCE: Fritz presentation, April 18, 2025.

THE ROLE OF ARTIFICIAL INTELLIGENCE AND NATURAL LANGUAGE PROCESSING IN CHRONIC PAIN AND DISABILITY DETERMINATIONS

V. G. Vinod Vydiswaran spoke about the use of artificial intelligence and medical natural language processing (NLP) to extract information from clinical notes in electronic health records (EHRs) that could be helpful for finding those at risk for high-impact chronic pain. In general, he explained, these data extraction methods are looking for computable phenotypes, or key characteristics about a patient that can be derived computationally, in the massive amount of data in an EHR. One study he and his collaborators conducted used NLP to identify risky alcohol use from clinical notes. In this study, NLP identified three times more patients with risky alcohol use than had been identified with International Classification of Diseases codes (Vydiswaran et al., 2024). NLP identified 87 percent true positives versus the 29 percent identified by International Classification of Diseases codes, the existing standard approach. Vydiswaran said researchers have developed NLP-based methods for extracting information from the EHR on social determinants of health, including alcohol use, tobacco use, drug use, and employment status, as well as disease state, medication use, and changes in those over time (Lybarger et al., 2023). In particular, deep neural network models have proven better at extracting this type of information than traditional machine learning–based models.

TABLE 8-1 Lessons Learned Partnering with Federally Qualified Health Centers

	Issues Encountered	Facilitators Identified	Strategies Implemented
Patient Access to Care	• Less predictable work hours • Multi-generational homes or housing instability • Limited tech for video visits	• Mobile phones are common • Respect for participants' time, being flexible, builds trust	• Offer sessions outside regular work hours • Flexible, non-judgmental (re)/scheduling
Adaptations to PT Interventions	• Limited community resources for physical activity • More likely to experience social stressors	• mHealth resources are available to support patients • Interventions for active coping with relaxation, mindfulness amenable to telehealth delivery	• Integrate mHealth to support education and exercise interventions • Integrate cognitive behavioral techniques
Patient-PT Working Alliance	• Remote delivery, language, culture are challenges in developing a working alliance	• Motivational interviewing is effective for building self-efficacy for behavior change using telehealth	• Train PTs in motivation and problem-solving (MAPS) treatment strategies
Culturally Competent Care	• Patients and PTs often have different cultural backgrounds • Patients' pain beliefs and coping preferences may be mismatched to evidence-based principles	• Care that respects participants' cultural perspectives helps build trust in PT • MAPS delivery can reduce risk for implicit bias from provider	• Train PTs in cultural competencies and awareness of their own cultural background • Training in person-centered MAPS delivery

NOTES: mHealth = mobile health; PT = physical therapy.
SOURCE: Fritz presentation, April 18, 2025.

Vydiswaran noted that chronic pain has been described in EHRs using structured data, such as pain intensity, treatment modalities, diagnostic codes, and interventions. Methods using these data, however, can only identify upward of 80 percent of individuals with chronic pain. In addition, while large language models have improved significantly in recent years, biased data, such as clinicians' dismissal of Black women's pain in clinical notes, beget biased models. There is active research on developing validated intersectionality-aware artificial intelligence models that can determine phenotypes such as pain.

9

Complementary and Alternative Therapies in Comprehensive Chronic Pain Management

The workshop's seventh session explored alternative and complementary pain treatments for chronic pain, the efficacy of those treatments, and how they can be integrated into conventional pain care to enhance physical, social, and psychological outcomes. The speakers were Tom Norris, retired Air Force lieutenant colonel and patient advisor with the American Chronic Pain Association; Peter Wayne, associate professor of medicine at Harvard Medical School and associate epidemiologist at Brigham and Women's Hospital; Richard Harris, Susan Samueli Endowed Chair and professor at the University of California, Irvine; and Anna Woodbury, associate professor and vice chair of research in the Department of Anesthesiology at Emory University School of Medicine.

THE COMPLEMENTARY AND INTEGRATIVE PAIN MANAGEMENT TOOLBOX

Tom Norris, who retired from the Air Force after treatment for testicular cancer that led to chronic pain, has been living with chronic pain for 37 years. Through multiple failed surgeries and a decade using fentanyl, which he successfully tapered off of, Norris found purpose and support by connecting with others, facilitating support groups, and advocating for patient-centered care.

Norris discussed the complementary and integrative pain management (CIPM) toolbox developed by the Alliance to Advance Comprehensive Integrative Pain Management (2022; Figure 9-1). Comprehensive care, he said, should include physical, psychological, social, spiritual, and lifestyle

47

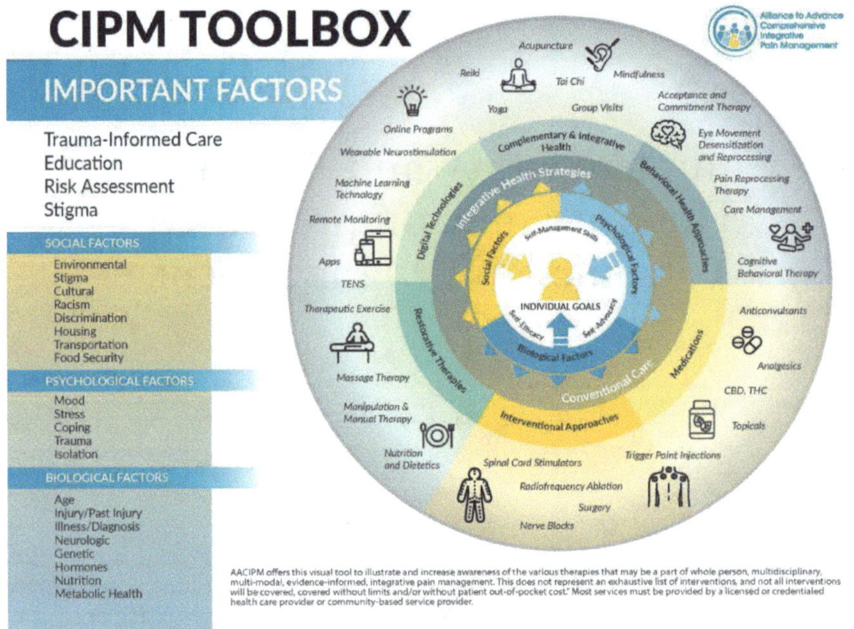

FIGURE 9-1 The complementary and integrative pain management toolbox.
SOURCES: Norris presentation, April 18, 2025; Pain Management Best Practices Inter-Agency Task Force, 2019.

elements. Though insurance does not cover all of these therapies, they still matter and can help someone live with chronic pain. He noted that most people living with chronic pain are unaware of all the components of effective pain control. Moreover, they struggle to be believed, cannot work, and are denied recognition and insurance coverage because they are living with a terrible, stigmatizing, and invisible disease.

When dealing with his chronic pain, Norris said he tried almost everything. The challenge, said Norris, is that the Social Security Administration (SSA) may recognize some therapies, such as epidural injections and psychotherapy, but others, such as journaling, virtual reality, and peer support, often are not recognized, even when they help people function, and only when they are formally prescribed or documented in the medical record.

Norris listed several barriers to achieving effective pain management. Complementary and alternative medicine therapies, for example, often go undocumented in medical records, while insurance rarely covers non-opioid options. Fragmented provider communication is another barrier. He noted the SSA disability system faces unique challenges given that chronic pain is often invisible, and treatment approaches such as yoga or pacing may be misread as full ability. Complementary and alternative medicine are often unrecognized unless formally prescribed, and people may fear reporting progress, worrying that doing so could jeopardize their benefits.

One model that works is the Veterans Administration (VA) Whole Health approach, which integrates complementary and alternative medicine therapies as core pain management tools. The Whole Health model empowers veterans to lead their care using evidence-informed and patient-centered treatments. He wondered if SSA could adopt similar approaches, such as acupuncture, massage therapy, mindfulness, biofeedback, tai chi, or yoga. He noted that when a system listens to science and lived experience, patients benefit.

Norris's take-home messages for SSA were that chronic pain is real, complex, and personal, with everyone feeling and interpreting pain differently. Effective communication is one important key to effective pain management, while validation and compassion are powerful support tools. The best care, he said, is flexible and accessible, and SSA should support—not penalize—people using complementary and alternative approaches to manage their chronic pain.

MINDFUL MOVEMENT FOR CHRONIC PAIN

Chronic pain, said Peter Wayne, is a complex condition best viewed as a biopsychosocial challenge affecting the body, mind, and social engagement (Dueñas et al., 2016); mindful movement interventions such as tai chi, yoga, and contemplative dance can help address each of its facets. Mindful movement, he explained, is distinct from conventional exercise and seated meditation. Rather, it is a form of movement or body positioning that includes a cleared state of mind, with the goal of achieving deep states of relaxation and breathing (Larkey et al., 2009) and heightened body and psychophysiological awareness (Osypiuk et al., 2018). Mindful movement, said Wayne, is best viewed from an embodied cognition framework in which mental and physical experiences co-create one another (Schmalzl and Kerr, 2016; Osypiuk et al., 2018).

Mind-body movement practices such as tai chi, said Wayne, are multi-modal, biopsychosocial mode-informed interventions with multiple components (Figure 9-2; Wayne and Fuerst, 2013). These components stimulate musculoskeletal tissues through movement and diverse postures while heightening somatic attention and mental focus. Imagery, visualization, breathing, autonomic regulation, higher level cognitive strategies such as kindness and self-gratitude, and psychosocial and physical interactions combine to enhance physical and psychosocial function, producing greater

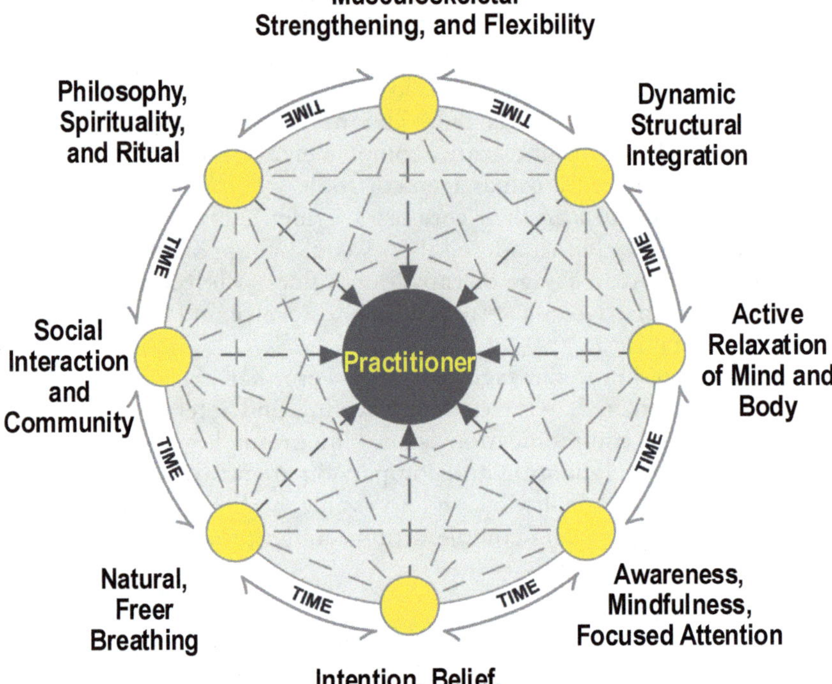

FIGURE 9-2 Multiple components of a biopsychosocially informed intervention for chronic pain.
SOURCES: Wayne presentation, April 18, 2025; Wayne and Fuerst, 2013. Copyright © 2013 by Harvard Health Publications. Reprinted by arrangement with The Permissions Company, LLC on behalf of Shambhala Publications Inc., Boulder, CO, shambhala.com.

interoceptive and exteroceptive acuity, healthier pain appraisal skills, and enhanced safety, self-efficacy, and adherence. Taken together, the end result is reduced pain and pain interference, said Wayne.

With more than 3,000 peer-reviewed articles on tai chi and qigong alone, the evidence supporting this approach to pain management is growing. One review he and his colleagues conducted of 210 systematic reviews of controlled trials, for example, found that "Tai Chi has multidimensional effects, including physical, psychological and quality of life benefits for a wide range of conditions, as well as multimorbidity. Clinically important benefits were most consistently reported for Parkinson's disease, falls risk, knee osteoarthritis, and cerebrovascular and cardiovascular disease including hypertension" (Yang et al., 2022).

Wayne reviewed a wide range of studies pertaining to the benefits of tai chi/qigong (TCQ) for several chronic musculoskeletal pain conditions. One review of 16 randomized controlled trials of TCQ for knee osteoarthritis found, for example, that TCQ produced improvements in pain and physical function that were greater than passive approaches (Kelley et al., 2022); another study comparing the effectiveness of TCQ versus physical therapy for knee osteoarthritis found that tai chi and physical therapy both improve pain and function scores, but only tai chi produced improvements on depression (Wang et al., 2016). Studies have also shown TCQ and meditation were helpful at managing low back pain (Yang et al., 2024) and neck pain (Lauche et al., 2016; Kong et al., 2022). Interoception—the body's ability to sense and interpret signals from within and provide awareness of internal states such as hunger, thirst, pain, and emotions—is a key mechanism linking mind-body practices and pain management, said Wayne (Voss et al., 2023).

Wayne said that mindful movement interventions are promising for reducing pain and disability across multiple musculoskeletal conditions, though more high-quality randomized controlled trials are warranted. It is unclear, for example, whether mindful movement interventions are more efficacious or safer than conventional exercises. Heightened body awareness and affective attention may enhance somatosensation and pain appraisal, which may then mediate clinical benefits directly through biomechanical efficiency, for example, and indirectly via safety, enjoyability, adherence, and mood. Larger studies powered for mediation analysis, factorial trial designs, and mechanistic studies are needed to inform relevance of top-down versus bottom-up training components.

ACUPUNCTURE AND ACUPRESSURE FOR CHRONIC PAIN

Richard Harris noted that more people live with chronic pain than with cancer, heart disease, and diabetes combined, with an estimated cost of $635 billion in the United States. It is one of the major reasons for individuals to try integrative medicine, including acupuncture, meditation, and TCQ, cited Harris. He noted the share of U.S. adults who used integrative health therapies increased from 19.2 percent in 2002 to 36.7 percent in 2022 (Nahin et al., 2024). Acupuncture as a treatment for pain rose from approximately 55 percent of individuals experiencing pain in 2002 to 73 percent in 2022, an increase that may have occurred because of insurance coverage for acupuncture and the availability of more studies showing efficacy (Nahin et al., 2024).

One of the early studies on the efficacy of acupuncture in managing pain showed the analgesic effect of acupuncture is greatest from several hours to two days after treatment, said Harris (Price et al., 1984). Studies have also shown that acupuncture significantly affects pain from migraines, osteoarthritis, and lower back and neck pain, with effect sizes that are larger than obtained with nonsteroidal anti-inflammatory agents (Vickers et al., 2012). Imaging studies have shown, too, that acupuncture deactivates the limbic system (Hui et al., 2000; Hui et al., 2005).

Though the evidence shows acupuncture is effective as a pain management technique, there are barriers to widespread adoption. One barrier is that many physicians do not know how to refer their patients to an acupuncturist. Harris said the National Certification Commission for Acupuncture and Oriental Medicine is a good place to start.[1] For individuals who do not live near a certified acupuncturist, Harris said there is an emerging body of evidence that self-acupressure using one's thumb might be effective for certain symptoms, including fatigue and sleep difficulties (Zick et al., 2016). Learning this technique takes approximately 15 minutes, he added. Harris and his colleagues have developed a self-acupressure smartphone app.

INTEGRATIVE SOLUTIONS FOR PAIN AND DISABILITY IN THE VETERANS ADMINISTRATION

U.S. veterans, said Anna Woodbury, experience higher rates and prevalence of chronic pain and more severe pain compared to nonveterans, with 9.1 percent of veterans living with severe pain (Taylor et al., 2024). She explained that integrative medicine combines conventional therapies, such as drugs and surgery, with complementary therapies, such as acupuncture and yoga. Since 2010 complementary and integrative health has been part of the VA's approach to treating pain in veterans, incorporating complementary evidence-based approaches such as massage therapy, acupuncture, mindfulness, tai chi, hypnosis, biofeedback, guided imagery, and yoga.[2] For example, evidence synthesized in 2023 showed that massage was likely to benefit veterans with chronic low back pain, fibromyalgia, and myofascial pain.

She noted the VA has implemented battlefield acupuncture, developed in 2001 to address acute and chronic pain, throughout its system. Battlefield acupuncture groups five acupuncture points on an individual's ear in a certain sequence capable of being deployed on the battlefield. A retrospective analysis involving more than 11,000 veterans found that over three-quarters of those treated experienced an immediate decrease in

---

[1] Available at www.nccaom.org (accessed May 13, 2025).

[2] VA Management briefs summarize the evidence supporting different complementary approaches the VA has adopted and are available at https://www.hsrd.research.va.gov/publications/management_briefs/default.cfm (accessed May 14, 2025).

pain, with an average decrease of 2.5 points (Zeliadt et al., 2020). This effect was smaller in veterans who had used opioids in the previous year. She noted that transauricular vagus nerve stimulation, which may operate on the same principle as battlefield acupuncture but uses a portable device that delivers mild electrical stimulation, is being developed to treat chronic pain (Patel et al., 2022). Certain VA centers also offer cranial electrotherapy stimulation, a device approved by the Food and Drug Administration for treating depression, anxiety, and insomnia, with some evidence showing it can decrease pain (Tan et al., 2011).

Woodbury said she hoped the rest of the U.S. health care system would follow the VA's lead and offer more complementary and integrative approaches to individuals living with chronic pain. In particular, she said, the public would benefit from battlefield acupuncture as an easy and rapid approach with proven benefits.

10

Emerging Research on New or Improved Methods for Measuring and Managing Chronic Pain

This session provided an overview of recent research on new or improved approaches to measuring and managing chronic pain. The speakers were Sean Mackey, Redlich Professor of anesthesiology, perioperative, and pain medicine, chief of the Division of Pain Medicine, and director of the Stanford Systems Neuroscience and Pain Lab at Stanford Medical School; Nathaniel Schuster, associate professor of anesthesiology at the University of California, San Diego; Konstantin Slavin, professor, chief of section, and fellowship director for stereotactic and functional neurosurgery in the Department of Neurosurgery at the University of Illinois Chicago; John Chae, executive vice president and chief academic officer for the MetroHealth System and professor of physical medicine and rehabilitation and biomedical engineering at Case Western Reserve University School of Medicine; Ming-Chih Jeffrey Kao, clinical associate professor of anesthesiology, perioperative, and pain medicine at the Stanford Pain Management Center; and Christin Veasley, pain research advocate and cofounder of the Chronic Pain Research Alliance.

THE FUTURE OF CHRONIC PAIN ASSESSMENT

Sean Mackey said patient-reported outcomes are the way researchers and clinicians typically measure pain, but the 0 to 10 pain intensity score is overly simplistic, is only moderately consistent, and does not account for a person's biopsychosocial, holistic aspects. What is needed, said Mackey, is a better way of capturing daily fluctuations in pain, tools reflecting the true lived experiences of those with chronic pain, and approaches to integrate the patient's perspective with objective measures.

Mackey noted there are different types of biomarkers, including diagnostic, predictive, prognostic, and safety (Figure 10-1; Mackey et al., 2019). Researchers are developing multi-omic biomarkers that use genetic, proteomic, metabolomic, and others, but none have yet been established as reliable biomarkers of chronic pain. The hope is that biomarkers can someday distinguish between different types of pain—inflammatory versus neuropathic pain, for example—and predict which treatment will work best for a given individual. While this is an emerging area of research, it is one about which Social Security Administration (SSA) adjudicators will have to become knowledgeable.

Another active area of research is investigating whether wearable technology can accurately monitor pain. Changes in activity and sleep patterns, which many digital watches now measure, might be linked to pain. Mackey predicted there will likely be rapid advances in this area, given the necessary sensors are inexpensive and widely used. Such devices may be able to provide SSA with real-world evidence of pain's functional limitations. Studies

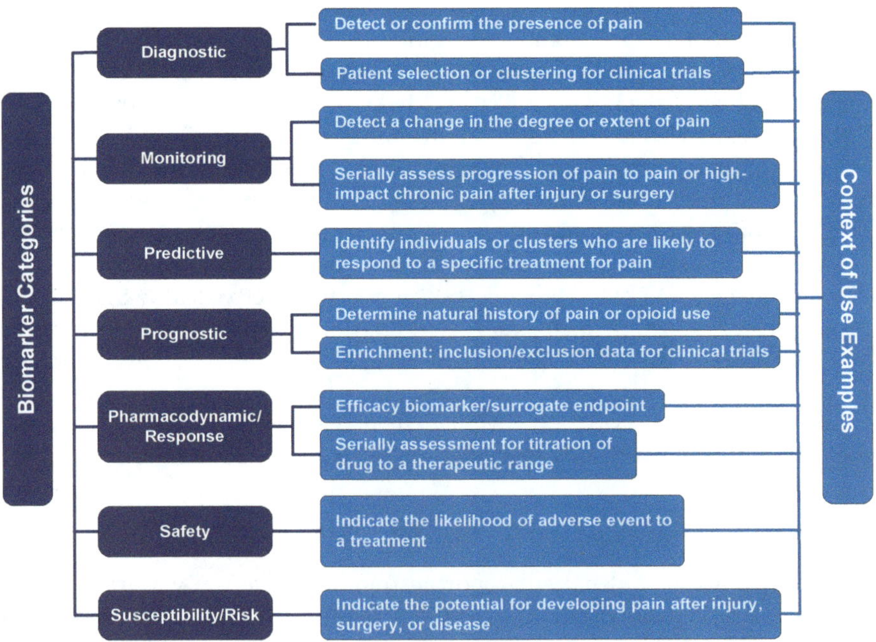

FIGURE 10-1 Pain biomarker categories and examples of their use.
SOURCES: Mackey presentation, April 18, 2025; Mackey et al., 2019. Copyright © 2019. Published by Wolters Kluwer Health, Inc. on behalf of The International Association for the Study of Pain. CC BY 4.0.

are also ongoing in quantitative sensory testing to measure pain thresholds and sensitivity, identify pain mechanisms, and match patients to targeted therapies. Quantitative sensory testing may be able to provide SSA with objective evidence of abnormal pain responses, noted Mackey.

Neuroimaging to visualize pain is one of the most interesting research areas to Mackey. Spinal cord and brain magnetic resonance imaging and positive emission tomography have produced pain signatures, while peripheral nerve imaging has identified pain sources. He noted that these methods are not yet at the point where they can tell if someone's pain is disabling, but research is heading in that direction (Davis et al., 2017).

What is clear is that no single biomarker will provide all the necessary information (Mackey et al., 2025). "It is not possible to completely encapsulate the experience of pain into one type of biomarker, and we need to fold these together," said Mackey. What is needed, he said, are composite, multimodal biomarker signatures, most likely enabled by artificial intelligence, to overcome the failure of electronic health records to integrate data and make them more actionable (Figure 10-2; Davis et al., 2020).

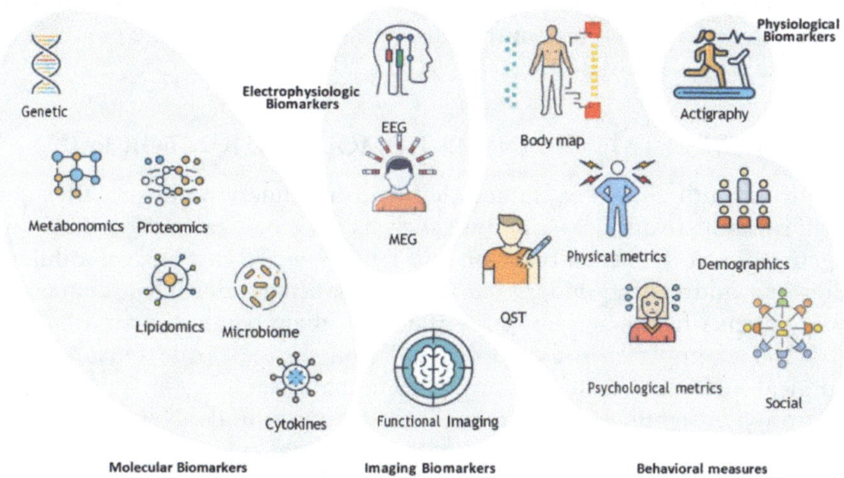

FIGURE 10-2 Composite, multimodal biomarker signatures for chronic pain. SOURCES: Mackey presentation, April 18, 2025; Mackey et al., 2025. Copyright © 2025, BMJ Publishing Group Ltd. on behalf of American Society of Regional Anesthesia & Pain Medicine. CC BY 4.0.

EMERGING PHARMACOTHERAPIES FOR
PAIN AND HEADACHE DISORDERS

Nathaniel Schuster discussed several emerging pharmacotherapy options for treating pain. He started with sodium channel inhibitors, the first of which the Food and Drug Administration (FDA) recently approved to treat moderate to severe acute pain. Sodium channel receptors, he explained, are highly expressed in pain-sensing neurons in the periphery and represent a drug target that might avoid central nervous system side effects.

Another class of drugs under development targets the transient receptor potential channels involved in pain sensation, explained Schuster. One drug candidate was well tolerated in a phase 1 clinical trial and is currently in a phase 2 study for acute migraine. Studies of a third class of molecules, known as Lyn tyrosine kinase inhibitors, have shown that they can reduce pain and are well tolerated (Tiecke et al., 2022).

Compounds found in marijuana, known as cannabinoids, may be useful as chronic pain treatments. Schuster noted that a 2017 report from the National Academies of Sciences, Engineering, and Medicine stated there was conclusive or substantial evidence that cannabis is effective for treating chronic pain in adults (NASEM, 2017). Psychedelic compounds, including LSD and psilocybin, are also the subject of pain treatment research and have shown some promise in treating certain types of chronic pain (Goel et al., 2023; Lyes et al., 2023; Askey et al., 2024).

DEVELOPMENTS IN NEUROMODULATION FOR PAIN

Konstantin Slavin explained that neuromodulation aims to alter nerve activity by delivering a stimulus, such as an electrical pulse or chemical agent, to restore normal function and relieve symptoms. Neuromodulation does not address the underlying problem causing pain, but it changes the way patients feel their symptoms and helps them regain function.

Today, implanting a neuromodulation device is the most common surgical intervention for treating chronic pain, said Slavin. These devices can provide significant pain reduction without opioids. Neuromodulation is customizable and adjustable and has minimal side effects compared to medications. Device implantation involves a minimally invasive procedure that can be reversed. FDA has approved a long list of devices, allowing clinicians the ability to select the right device for the right indications.

Slavin said a new direction in neuromodulation is looking at its utility outside of stimulating specific regions of the spinal cord. The newest devices can stimulate the dorsal root ganglion and treat complex regional pain syndromes (Deer et al., 2013). Burst-mode devices, which deliver pulsed rather than continuous stimulation, work on both the somatic pain system that localizes pain and the medial pain pathways involved in the emotional processing of pain (De Ridder et al., 2013). One limitation of this approach is that some people develop tolerance to the stimuli.

PERCUTANEOUS PERIPHERAL NERVE STIMULATION

John Chae discussed his work developing percutaneous peripheral nerve stimulation to treat shoulder pain after stroke. With electrodes anchored in the muscle surrounding a patient's shoulder, the nerve to the muscle is stimulated, causing it to contract and provide feedback to the central nervous system. This feedback is believed to modulate central sensitization. After 30 to 60 days, he removes the electrode, but the therapeutic effect—a significant reduction in shoulder pain—remains (Chae et al., 2005; Wilson et al., 2014).

Based on these results and others, Chae said that if central sensitization is the convergent mechanism behind chronic musculoskeletal pain in general, and if percutaneous peripheral nerve stimulation reduces shoulder pain via modulation of central sensitization, then percutaneous peripheral nerve stimulation should reduce musculoskeletal pain in general. In fact, a recent review of prospective studies concluded that percutaneous peripheral nerve stimulation for up to 60 days "provides durable clinically significant improvements in pain and pain interference. Similar efficacy across diverse targets and etiologies supports the broad applicability for use within the chronic pain population using this non-opioid technology" (Pritzlaff et al., 2024). Another recent "real-world" retrospective review found that 71 percent of over 6,000 patients experienced greater than 50 percent pain relief and improved quality of life (Huntoon et al., 2023). The device received FDA clearance in 2016 and has been placed in over 36,000 patients.

Chae also briefly discussed high-frequency blocks as a treatment for pain. This technique, which delivers high-frequency stimulation to block nerve impulses, was first developed to treat post-amputation pain and received FDA clearance in 2024 (Kapural et al., 2024).

EMERGING DIGITAL TECHNOLOGIES FOR MEASURING AND MANAGING CHRONIC PAIN

Ming-Chih Jeffrey Kao provided a high-level survey of emerging digital technologies for measuring and managing chronic pain. In 2023 FDA approved the first device for quantitative assessment of nociception during surgery. This device features a finger probe that gathers information on a patient's heart rate, skin moisture, movement, and temperature and produces a composite objective acute pain score. In a clinical trial, patients whose anesthesia was guided by this device received 30 percent less opioid pain medication during surgery and experienced fewer episodes of low blood pressure (Meijer et al., 2019). Kao noted that FDA's approval set a precedent for objective acute pain measurement devices, which should encourage further innovation.

Turning to the subject of pain management, Kao noted that in 2025, the Centers for Medicare & Medicaid Services began covering digital mental health treatment, a category of prescription digital therapeutics that require FDA clearance as a medical device. Digital mental health treatment has the potential, said Kao, to address the worsening health care worker shortage the United States faces over the next decade. Kao noted that disability-focused software is not eligible for FDA's Breakthrough Devices Program.

There are several digital therapeutic solutions for home physical therapy under development. A clinical trial of one such device found that an eight-week digital physical therapy program improved pain and pain interference in individuals with low back pain that was equivalent to conventional in-person physical therapy, though the digital group had half the dropout rate. Kao said the majority of digital rehabilitation therapeutics rely on advanced computer vision to detect the patient's movements using pose estimation algorithms (Stenum et al., 2024). He noted that none of the eight commonly used pose estimation algorithms were trained using data that included disabled individuals, though studies are ongoing to address this shortcoming.

Kao said virtual reality is also emerging as a powerful tool for pain management without pharmaceuticals. In a clinical trial, a 56-day virtual reality program comprising daily sessions lasting 2 to 16 minutes each produced significant reductions in pain intensity and pain interference in individuals with low back pain that lasted for up to 24 months (Maddox et al., 2023).

While promising alternatives to medication, Kao said hardware-based digital therapies face significant accessibility hurdles, including cost, physical usability challenges, and inconsistent insurance reimbursement. Addressing these barriers, he said, is crucial to achieving equitable access.

Kao discussed the use of large language models, such as ChatGPT, for summarizing information in electronic health records. In one recent study, ChatGPT 4.0 summaries of radiology reports, patient questions, progress notes, and doctor–patient dialogue were deemed to be either equivalent or superior compared with summaries from medical experts (Van Veen et al., 2024). In contrast, an earlier study using ChatGPT 3.5 found it was prone to generating incorrect summaries (Tang et al., 2023). The lesson here is that humans must be in the loop to ensure safety and accuracy. Kao noted that large language models can complement natural language processing and artificial intelligence systems by providing better context, summaries, and decision support.

CO-CREATING PAIN THERAPEUTICS:
WHERE INNOVATION MEETS LIVED EXPERIENCE

In her presentation, Christin Veasley addressed the reasons new therapeutics and innovation are needed for chronic pain treatment. She noted that deciding on treatment is complicated for an individual who lives with chronic pain, making it important that these decisions are made in partnership between clinician and patient. In making these decisions, factors such as the emotional toll, financial burden, and social impact are also involved.

Moreover, while there are many therapeutic options available, patients and clinicians alike have little or no evidence to guide them in making an informed decision, leading to a trial-and-error approach that can be costly, both financially and emotionally, and take an extreme physical toll. In her case, finding the right treatment for her chronic pain took 6 years with 6 clinicians, 20 to 25 hours a week, and tens of thousands of dollars a year trying dozens of medications and dozens of nonpharmacologic interventions. "I lost years of my life to 'let's see if this works,'" said Veasley.

An underappreciated aspect of this type of journey that many people living with chronic pain face is the complexity of the risk-benefit decisions they must make for every single treatment they try (Figure 10-3). "It is not just the efficacy; it is also about the side effects," said Veasley. Other considerations include how the treatment may impact a person's ability to function, the financial burden, insurance coverage, appointment scheduling, and recovery time.

Complicating these decisions further, said Veasley, is the fact that many people have multiple pain conditions or multisite body pain along with comorbidities such as sleep disorders, mood disorders, cognitive impairment, and fatigue. As a result, treatments often need to be multimodal, and a risk-benefit analysis goes into each aspect of a treatment plan. In addition, it's likely that people have other chronic diseases, since 6 in 10 U.S. adults have at least one chronic illness, and 4 in 10 have two or more. Treatment choices must then factor in heart disease or diabetes. "As you have more

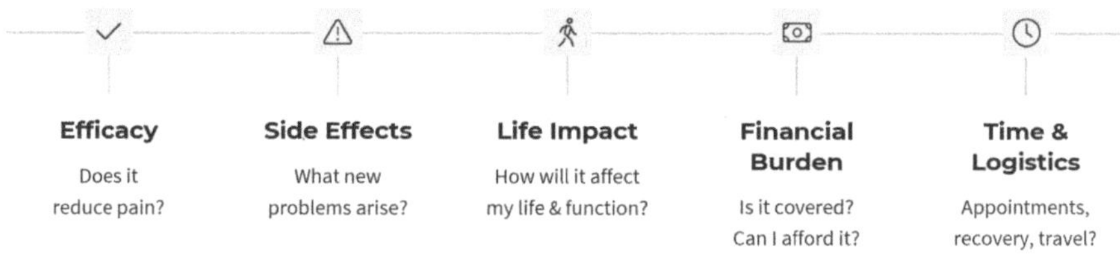

FIGURE 10-3 Real-world decision dilemmas make risk–benefit decisions complex.
SOURCE: Veasley presentation, April 18, 2025.

conditions or you are considering additional treatments, the decision tree grows exponentially," said Veasley. "Then we are in this place where it is almost impossible to weigh all the risks and benefits simultaneously to identify the best overall treatment plan."

The goal, said Veasley, is to end the trial-and-error era, and that requires better data to identify which treatments will work for which patients and to develop predictors of success. It also requires studying additive effects of treatment combinations and meaningful metrics to help individuals prioritize the outcomes that matter most to them. In addition, too many treatments have been evaluated only over the short term, with little grasp as to how they work over a person's lifetime.

Key to addressing all of these challenges and complexities will be to partner with patients throughout the entire research and development cycle, starting at the very beginning with designing new and innovative therapeutics that take patients' critical needs and input into consideration. This partnership should continue all the way through the research lifecycle, including patient-centered study design, execution of clinical trials, and implementation of new therapeutics (Haroutounian et al., 2024). "People are more likely to adopt solutions they help create, for that builds trust—a critical issue in the research landscape," said Veasley. Regarding development of novel diagnostics for chronic pain, she noted that while the goal of pain research is to garner objective data, the experience of chronic pain remains subjective, and patients' reports of their physical and emotional experiences should be prioritized. Also imperative is to design novel diagnostics and treatments that are accessible, non-intrusive, affordable, and easy for everyone to use.

11

Key Challenges and Opportunities in Chronic Pain and Disability

In the workshop's final session, planning committee members presented their key takeaways from sessions they moderated.

Session 1: Factors Affecting Access to Effective Chronic Pain Care (Tamara Baker, professor of psychiatry, University of North Carolina at Chapel Hill).

- Social and structural determinants of health must be considered by clinicians, researchers, and policy makers with regard to access to and availability of care and treatment.
- Age and race are important characteristics and must also be considered in future plans and next steps.

Session 2: Methods and Metrics for Chronic Pain Assessment in Adults and Children (Reuben Escorpizo, clinical professor, University of Vermont College of Nursing and Health Sciences).

- Pain is a multidimensional, individualized, biopsychosocial, and temporal experience.
- A biopsychosocial perspective on chronic pain is essential, requiring a holistic manner of assessment.
- Assessment requires observational, performance-based, and self-report measures that together are powerful tools for informing disability determination decisions.
- Challenges include standardizing both assessment and reporting for comparability and benchmarking.

- Patients must be an active part of the measurement and treatment development process.

Session 3: Best Practices and Clinical Perspectives on Chronic Pain Treatment and Management in Children (Henry Xiang, professor of pediatrics and epidemiology at the Ohio State University and director of the Center for Pediatric Trauma Research at Nationwide Children's Hospital).
- Data are critical for allocating resources, but there is a lack of comprehensive data on chronic pain experience, etiology, and treatment outcomes in children, and on the proportion of children with chronic pain who transition to adulthood with chronic pain.
- An important research question is how early intervention during childhood reduces the likelihood that an individual will file for disability claim as an adult.
- A triage system is needed to identify children who need treatment in the limited number of comprehensive treatment programs versus those who can receive treatment at a community hospital or primary care office.
- Research on innovative technologies must involve more patients and their families to ensure that the technologies are relevant and accessible.

Session 4: Best Practices on Chronic Pain Treatment and Management in Adults (Christopher Standaert, associate professor of physical medicine and rehabilitation services at the University of Pittsburgh School of Medicine).
- Effective chronic pain treatment focuses on improving the individual's quality of life in meaningful ways. However, this is difficult to achieve within the fragmented and financially driven U.S. health care system.
- Clinicians do not spend enough time talking to their patients about their lives, needs, and wants, and they do not explain the harms of possible treatments in a way that helps them decide on a course of action.
- Physical movement, physical capacity, and psychological well-being are central to chronic pain care and high levels of functioning.
- Within the U.S. health care system, there is a need to emphasize non-pharmacologic and noninvasive therapeutic options, such as tai chi and pain psychology, that are effective at treating chronic pain.

Session 5: Patient Journeys and Clinician Perspectives in Treating and Managing Chronic Pain (Anna Williams, vice president, Clusterbusters, and Juan Hincapie-Castillo, assistant professor of epidemiology at the University of North Carolina at Chapel Hill).

Anna Williams:
- Many people living with chronic pain experience grief, fear, and humiliation and feel helpless and unheard; there is a communication disconnect when patients don't understand medical jargon or fit into neat diagnostic categories.
- Patients value a sense of dignity, provider emphasis on quality of life, and empowerment with their choice of treatments.
- Stigma and health care disparities of care related to geographic location, race, age, and other factors impede effective management of chronic pain.
- Each individual experiences chronic pain differently.

Juan Hincapie-Castillo:
- Limited continuity of care and care coordination among providers creates significant challenges for underserved and uninsured populations.
- Those living in rural areas face challenges accessing effective complementary and alternative therapies.
- The lack of physicians trained in pain management creates opportunities for collaboration with other clinicians, such as clinical pharmacists.
- Clinicians receive insufficient training in pain management and disability claim criteria.
- Doctor shopping, which can be a concern for Social Security disability adjudicators, could be a reflection of patients facing discrimination in their care and advocating for themselves to get the care they need.
- Even when chronic pain is controlled, significant impairment and disability can persist, which creates challenges for Social Security disability adjudicators.

Sessions 6 and 7: Health Care System Challenges in Comprehensive Chronic Pain Management, and Complementary and Alternative Therapies in Comprehensive Chronic Pain Management (Kim Dupree Jones, professor and associate dean for academic advancement at Emory University).
- Chronic pain is multisymptomatic, requiring measurement of multiple domains to determine the most appropriate treatment options.
- Physical therapy, home exercise, and mindful movement are evidence-based, effective therapies that improve pain, reduce fatigue, and improve sleep, and the U.S. health care system needs to more readily adopt them.

Session 8: Emerging Research on New or Improved Methods for Measuring and Managing Chronic Pain (Sean Mackey, Redlich Professor of anesthesiology, perioperative, and pain medicine, chief of the division of pain medicine, and director of the Stanford Systems Neuroscience and Pain Lab at Stanford Medical School).

- New interventions, including medications, neuromodulation, and mind-body approaches, are in development, but there is a need to accelerate the pipeline from idea to implementation.
- The research community needs to provide higher-quality data to help the Social Security Administration streamline the disability application and determination process.
- To obtain the required data, clinicians must be equipped with improved methods for capturing them, which includes financial incentives that align with this goal.

References

Alaiti, R. K., J. Castro, H. Lee, J. P. Caneiro, J. W. S. Vlaeyen, S. J. Kamper, and M. F. da Costa. 2022. What are the mechanisms of action of cognitive-behavioral, mind-body, and exercise-based interventions for pain and disability in people with chronic primary musculoskeletal pain? A systematic review of mediation studies from randomized controlled trials. *The Journal of Clinical Pain* 38(7):502–509.

Alliance to Advance Comprehensive Integrative Pain Management. 2022. Comprehensive and Integrative Pain Management Toolbox. August. https://painmanagementalliance.org/what-iscipm/ (accessed June 26, 2025).

Ardito, R. B., and D. Rabellino. 2011. Therapeutic alliance and outcome of psychotherapy: Historical excursus, measurements, and prospects for research. *Frontiers in Psychology* 2:270.

Aroke, E. N., P. V. Joseph, A. Roy, D. S. Overstreet, T. O. Tollefsbol, D. E. Vance, and B. R. Goodin. 2019. Could epigenetics help explain racial disparities in chronic pain? *Journal of Pain Research* 12:701–710.

Aroke, E. N., P. Jackson, L. Meng, Z. Huo, D. S. Overstreet, T. M. Penn, T. L. Quinn, Y. Cruz-Almeida, and B. R. Goodin. 2022a. Differential DNA methylation in Black and White individuals with chronic low back pain enrich different genomic pathways. *Neurobiology of Pain* 11:100086.

Aroke, E. N., J. M. Hobson, T. Ptacek, P. Jackson, and B. R. Goodin. 2022b. Genome-wide DNA methylation study identifies significant epigenomic changes associated with internalized stigma in adults with non-specific chronic low back pain. *Frontiers in Pain Research (Lausanne)* 3.

Askey, T., R. Lasrado, M. Maiarú, and G. J. Stephens. 2024. Psilocybin as a novel treatment for chronic pain. *British Journal of Pharmacology* 1–14. https://doi.org/10.1111/bph.17420.

Balba, N. M., A. A. McBride, M. L. Callahan, S. D. Mist, K. D. Jones, M. P. Butler, M. M. Lim, and M. M. Heinricher. 2022. Photosensitivity is associated with chronic pain following traumatic brain injury. *Journal of Neurotrauma* 39(17–18):1183–1194.

Barhorst, E. E., A. E. Boruch, D. B. Cook, and J. B. Lindheimer. 2021. Pain-related post-exertional malaise in myalgic encephalomyelitis / chronic fatigue syndrome (ME/CFS) and fibromyalgia: A systematic review and three-level meta-analysis. *Pain Medicine* 23(6):1144–1157.

Bartley, E. J., N. I. Hossain, C. C. Gravlee, K. T. Sibille, E. L. Terry, I. A. Vaughn, J. S. Cardoso, S. Q. Booker, T. L. Glover, B. R. Goodin, A. Sotolongo, K. A. Thompson, H. W. Bulls, R. Staud, J. C. Edberg, L. A. Bradley, and R. B. Fillingim. 2019. Race/ethnicity moderates the association between psychosocial resilience and movement-evoked pain in knee osteoarthritis. *ACR Open Rheumatology* 1(1):16–25.

Booker, S. Q., and T. Okolie. 2024. Pain-affirming care at the intersection of race, aging, and pain management nursing. *Pain Management Nursing* 25(4):323–326.

Borsook, D., and E. Kalso. 2013. Transforming pain medicine: Adapting to science and society. *European Journal of Pain* 17(8). https://doi.org/10.1002/j.1532-2149.2013.00297.

Chae, J., D. T. Yu, M. E. Walker, A. Kirsteins, E. P. Elovic, S. R. Flanagan, R. L. Harvey, R. D. Zorowitz, F. S. Frost, J. H. Grill, and Z.-P. Fang. 2005. Intramuscular electrical stimulation for hemiplegic shoulder pain: A 12-month follow-up of a multiple-center, randomized clinical trial. *American Journal of Physical Medicine & Rehabilitation* 84(11):832–842.

Chambers, C. T., J. Dol, P. R. Tutelman, C. L. Langley, J. A. Parker, B. T. Cormier, G. J. Macfarlane, G. T. Jones, D. Chapman, N. Proudfoot, A. Grant, and J. Marianayagam. 2024. The prevalence of chronic pain in children and adolescents: A systematic review update and meta-analysis. *Pain* 165(10):2215–2234.

Chronic Pain Research Alliance. 2023. *About COPCs.* https://chronicpainresearch.org/about_copcs/ (accessed July 18, 2025).

Choy, E., S. Perrot, T. Leon, J. Kaplan, D. Petersel, A. Ginovker, and E. Kramer. 2010. A patient survey of the impact of fibromyalgia and the journey to diagnosis. *BMC Health Services Research* 10:102.

Clauw, D. J., M. N. Essex, V. Pitman, and K. D. Jones. 2019. Reframing chronic pain as a disease, not a symptom: Rationale and implications for pain management. *Postgraduate Medicine* 131(3):185–198.

Darnall, B. 2019. *Psychological treatments for patients with chronic pain.* Washington, DC: American Psychological Association.

Darnall, B. D. 2025a. Brief interventions for chronic pain: Approaches and evidence. *Current Opinion in Psychology* 62:101978.

Darnall, B. D. 2025b. Empowering pain relief. *ASA Monitor* 89(3).

Darnall, B. D., J. Scheman, S. Davin, J. W. Burns, J. L. Murphy, A. C. Wilson, R. D. Kerns, and S. C. Mackey. 2016. Pain psychology: A global needs assessment and national call to action. *Pain Medicine* 17(2):250–263.

Darnall, B. D., A. Roy, A. L. Chen, M. S. Ziadni, R. T. Keane, D. S. You, K. Slater, H. Poupore-King, I. Mackey, M.-C. Kao, K. F. Cook, K. Lorig, D. Zhang, J. Hong, L. Tian, and S. C. Mackey. 2021. Comparison of a single-session pain management skills intervention with a single-session health education intervention and 8 sessions of cognitive behavioral therapy in adults with chronic low back pain: A randomized clinical trial. *JAMA Network Open* 4(8):e2113401.

Darnall, B. D., K. A. Edwards, R. E. Courtney, M. S. Ziadni, L. E. Simons, and L. E. Harrison. 2023. Innovative treatment formats, technologies, and clinician trainings that improve access to behavioral pain treatment for youth and adults. *Frontiers in Pain Research (Lausanne)* 4.

Darnall, B. D., J. W. Burns, J. Hong, A. Roy, K. Slater, H. Poupore-King, M. S. Ziadni, D. S. You, C. Jung, K. F. Cook, K. Lorig, L. Tian, and S. C. Mackey. 2024. Empowered Relief, cognitive behavioral therapy, and health education for people with chronic pain: A comparison of outcomes at 6-month follow-up for a randomized controlled trial. *Pain Reports* 9(1):e1116.

Davin, S. A., J. Savage, N. R. Thompson, A. Schuster, and B. D. Darnall. 2022. Transforming standard of care for spine surgery: Integration of an online single-session behavioral pain management class for perioperative optimization. *Frontiers in Pain Research (Lausanne)* 3:856252.

Davis, K. D., H. Flor, H. T. Greely, G. D. Iannetti, S. Mackey, M. Ploner, A. Pustilnik, I. Tracey, R. D. Treede, and T. D. Wager. 2017. Brain imaging tests for chronic pain: Medical, legal and ethical issues and recommendations. *Nature Reviews Neurology* 13(10):624–638.

Davis, K. D., N. Aghaeepour, A. H. Ahn, M. S. Angst, D. Borsook, A. Brenton, M. E. Burczynski, C. Crean, R. Edwards, B. Gaudilliere, G. W. Hergenroeder, M. J. Iadarola, S. Iyengar, Y. Jiang, J. T. Kong, S. Mackey, C. Y. Saab, C. N. Sang, J. Scholz, M. Segerdahl, I. Tracey, C. Veasley, J. Wang, T. D. Wager, A. D. Wasan, and M. A. Pelleymounter. 2020. Discovery and validation of biomarkers to aid the development of safe and effective pain therapeutics: Challenges and opportunities. *Nature Reviews Neurology* 16(7):381–400.

Deer, T. R., E. Grigsby, R. L. Weiner, B. Wilcosky, and J. M. Kramer. 2013. A prospective study of dorsal root ganglion stimulation for the relief of chronic pain. *Neuromodulation* 16(1):67–71.

Delitto, A., C. G. Patterson, J. M. Stevans, J. K. Freburger, S. S. Khoja, M. J. Schneider, C. M. Greco, J. A. Freel, G. A. Sowa, A. D. Wasan, G. P. Brennan, S. J. Hunter, K. I. Minick, S. T. Wegener, P. L. Ephraim, J. M. Beneciuk, S. Z. George, and R. B. Saper. 2021. Stratified care to prevent chronic low back pain in high-risk patients: The TARGET trial. A multi-site pragmatic cluster randomized trial. *EClinicalMedicine* 34:100795.

De Ridder, D., M. Plazier, N. Kamerling, T. Menovsky, and S. Vanneste. 2013. Burst spinal cord stimulation for limb and back pain. *World Neurosurgery* 80(5):642–649.e1.

Dueñas, M., B. Ojeda, A. Salazar, J. A. Mico, and I. Failde. 2016. A review of chronic pain impact on patients, their social environment and the health care system. *Journal of Pain Research* 9:457–467.

Durbhakula, S., T. Y. Wang, K. G. Segna, G. R. Limerick, M. Y. Broachwala, M. E. Schatman, M. A. Zaidi, I. J. Siddarthan, and S. Toy. 2024. Shifts in students' attitudes towards pain patients, pain, and opioid management following a dedicated medical school pain curriculum. *Journal of Pain Research* 2(17):827–835. https:/doi.org/10.2147/JPR.S447671.

Evans, J. R., E. Benore, and G. A. Banez. 2016. The cost-effectiveness of intensive inter-disciplinary pediatric chronic pain rehabilitation. *Journal of Pediatric Psychology* 41(8):849–856.

Farrokhi, S., E. Russell Esposito, D. McPherson, B. Mazzone, R. Condon, C. G. Patterson, M. Schneider, C. M. Greco, A. Delitto, M. J. Highsmith, B. D. Hendershot, J. Maikos, and C. L. Dearth. 2020. Resolving the Burden of Low Back Pain in Military Service Members and Veterans (RESOLVE): Protocol for a multisite pragmatic clinical trial. *Pain Medicine* 21(Suppl 2):s45–s52.

Firestone, K. A., H. Johnston, J. Portanova, and K. D. Jones. 2025. Integrating complex pain concepts into prelicensure nursing education: An unfolding case study to enhance clinical reasoning and competency. *Nurse Educator* 50(3):165–168.

Fisher, E., E. Law, J. Dudeney, T. M. Palermo, G. Stewart, and C. Eccleston. 2018. Psychological therapies for the management of chronic and recurrent pain in children and adolescents. *Cochrane Database of Systematic Reviews* 9(9):Cd003968.

Freij, K. W., F. Agbor, K. R. Kinnie, V. Srinivasasainagendra, T. L. Quinn, H. K. Tiwari, R. E. Sorge, B. R. Goodin, and E. N. Aroke. 2024. The pace of biological aging significantly mediates the relationship between internalized stigma of chronic pain and chronic low back pain severity among non-Hispanic black but not non-Hispanic white adults. *Neurobiology of Pain* 16:100170.

Friedrichsdorf, S. J., A. Postier, D. Eull, C. Weidner, L. Foster, M. Gilbert, and F. Campbell. 2015. Pain outcomes in a US children's hospital: A cross-sectional survey. *Hospital Pediatrics* 5(1):18–26.

Friedrichsdorf, S. J., J. Giordano, K. Desai Dakoji, A. Warmuth, C. Daughtry, and C. A. Schulz. 2016. Chronic pain in children and adolescents: Diagnosis and treatment of primary pain disorders in head, abdomen, muscles and joints. *Children (Basel)* 3(4).

Friend, R., R. M. Bennett, J. H. Aebischer, A. W. St. John, and K. D. Jones. 2021. Validating the revised Symptom Impact Questionnaire with a proposed fibromyalgia phenotype using experimentally-induced pain and patient self-reports. *Clinical and Experimental Rheumatology* 39 Suppl 130(3):137–143.

Gatchel, R. J., and K. H. Rollings. 2008. Evidence-informed management of chronic low back pain with cognitive behavioral therapy. *The Spine Journal* 8(1):40–44.

George, S. Z., and M. D. Bishop. 2018. Chronic musculoskeletal pain is a nervous system disorder... Now what? *Physical Therapy* 98(4):209–213.

Goel, A., Y. Rai, S. Sivadas, C. Diep, H. Clarke, H. Shanthanna, and K. S. Ladha. 2023. Use of psychedelics for pain: A scoping review. *Anesthesiology* 139(4):523–536.

Greco, C. M., S. A. Gaylord, K. Faurot, J. M. Weinberg, P. Gardiner, I. Roth, J. L. Barnhill, H. N. Thomas, S. C. Dhamne, C. Lathren, J. E. Baez, S. Lawrence, T. Neogi, K. E. Lasser, M. G. Castro, A. M. White, S. J. Simmons, C. Ferrao, D. D. Binda, N. Elhadidy, K. M. Eason, K. M. McTigue, and N. E. Morone. 2021. The design and methods of the OPTIMUM study: A multisite pragmatic randomized clinical trial of a telehealth group mindfulness program for persons with chronic low back pain. *Contemporary Clinical Trials* 109:106545.

Griffin, A., L. Wilson, A. B. Feinstein, A. Bortz, M. S. Heirich, R. Gilkerson, J. F. Wagner, M. Menendez, T. J. Caruso, S. Rodriguez, S. Naidu, B. Golianu, and L. E. Simons. 2020. Virtual reality in pain rehabilitation for youth with chronic pain: Pilot feasibility study. *JMIR Rehabilitation Assistive Technologies* 7(2):e22620.

Groenewald, C. B., B. S. Essner, D. Wright, M. D. Fesinmeyer, and T. M. Palermo. 2014. The economic costs of chronic pain among a cohort of treatment-seeking adolescents in the United States. *The Journal of Pain* 15(9):925–933.

Groenewald, C. B., D. R. Wright, and T. M. Palermo. 2015. Health care expenditures associated with pediatric pain-related conditions in the United States. *Pain* 156(5):951–957.

Haroutounian, S., K. J. Holzer, R. D. Kerns, C. Veasley, R. H. Dworkin, D. C. Turk, K. L. Carman, C. T. Chambers, P. Cowan, R. R. Edwards, J. C. Eisenach, J. T. Farrar, M. Ferguson, L. P. Forsythe, R. Freeman, J. S. Gewandter, I. Gilron, C. Goertz, H. Grol-Prokopczyk, S. Iyengar, I. Jordan, C. Kamp, B. A. Kleykamp, R. L. Knowles, D. J. Langford, S. Mackey, R. Malamut, J. Markman, K. R. Martin, E. McNicol, K. V. Patel, A. S. C. Rice, M. Rowbotham, F. Sandbrink, L. S. Simon, D. J. Steiner, and J. Vollert. 2024. Patient engagement in designing, conducting, and disseminating clinical pain research: IMMPACT recommended considerations. *Pain* 165(5):1013–1028.

Hayden, J. A., J. Ellis, R. Ogilvie, A. Malmivaara, and M. W. van Tulder. 2021. Exercise therapy for chronic low back pain. *Cochrane Database of Systematic Reviews* 9(9):Cd009790.

Heathcote, L. C., J. Rabner, A. Lebel, J. M. Hernandez, and L. E. Simons. 2018. Rapid screening of risk in pediatric headache: Application of the pediatric pain screening tool. *Journal of Pediatric Psychology* 43(3):243–251.

Higgins, K. S., K. A. Birnie, C. T. Chambers, A. C. Wilson, L. Caes, A. J. Clark, M. Lynch, J. Stinson, and M. Campbell-Yeo. 2015. Offspring of parents with chronic pain: A systematic review and meta-analysis of pain, health, psychological, and family outcomes. *Pain* 156(11):2256–2266.

Hoffman, K. M., S. Trawalter, J. R. Axt, and M. N. Oliver. 2016. Racial bias in pain assessment and treatment recommendations, and false beliefs about biological differences between Blacks and Whites. *Proceedings of the National Academy of Sciences of the United States of America* 113(16):4296–4301.

Huguet, A., and J. Miró. 2008. The severity of chronic pediatric pain: An epidemiological study. *The Journal of Pain* 9(3):226–236.

Hui, K. K., J. Liu, N. Makris, R. L. Gollub, A. J. Chen, C. I. Moore, D. N. Kennedy, B. R. Rosen, and K. K. Kwong. 2000. Acupuncture modulates the limbic system and subcortical gray structures of the human brain: Evidence from fMRI studies in normal subjects. *Human Brain Mapping* 9(1):13–25.

Hui, K. K., J. Liu, O. Marina, V. Napadow, C. Haselgrove, K. K. Kwong, D. N. Kennedy, and N. Makris. 2005. The integrated response of the human cerebro-cerebellar and limbic systems to acupuncture stimulation at ST 36 as evidenced by fMRI. *NeuroImage* 27(3):479–496.

Huntoon, M. A., K. V. Slavin, J. M. Hagedorn, N. D. Crosby, and J. W. Boggs. 2023. A retrospective review of real-world outcomes following 60-day peripheral nerve stimulation for the treatment of chronic pain. *Pain Physician* 26(3):273–281.

Johnson, A. J., T. Vasilopoulos, S. Q. Booker, J. Cardoso, E. L. Terry, K. Powell-Roach, R. Staud, D. A. Kusko, A. S. Addison, D. T. Redden, B. R. Goodin, R. B. Fillingim, and K. T. Sibille. 2021. Knee pain trajectories over 18 months in non-Hispanic Black and non-Hispanic White adults with or at risk for knee osteoarthritis. *BMC Musculoskeletal Disorders* 22(1):415.

Jones, K. D., L. A. King, S. D. Mist, R. M. Bennett, and F. B. Horak. 2011. Postural control deficits in people with fibromyalgia: A pilot study. *Arthritis Research & Therapy* 13(4):R127.

Jones, M. D., H. J. Hansford, A. Bastianon, M. T. Gibbs, Y. L. Gilanyi, N. E. Foster, S. G. Dean, R. Ogilvie, J. A. Hayden, and L. Wood. 2025. Exercise adherence is associated with improvements in pain intensity and functional limitations in adults with chronic non-specific low back pain: A secondary analysis of a Cochrane review. *Journal of Physiotherapy* 71(2):91–99.

Kapos, F. P., K. D. Craig, S. R. Anderson, S. F. Bernardes, A. T. Hirsh, K. Karos, E. Keogh, E. A. Reynolds Losin, J. L. McParland, D. J. Moore, and C. E. Ashton-James. 2024. Social determinants and consequences of pain: Toward multilevel, intersectional, and life course perspectives. *The Journal of Pain* 25(10).

Kapural, L., B. Kim, J. Eidt, E. A. Petersen, J. M. Schwalb, K. V. Slavin, and N. Mekhail. 2024. Long-term treatment of chronic postamputation pain with bioelectric nerve block: Twelve-month results of the randomized, double-blinded, cross-over QUEST study. *Neuromodulation* 27(8):1383–1392.

Kelley, G. A., K. S. Kelley, and L. F. Callahan. 2022. Clinical relevance of tai chi on pain and physical function in adults with knee osteoarthritis: An ancillary meta-analysis of randomized controlled trials. *Science Progress* 105(2):368504221088375.

Knoebel, R. W., J. V. Starck, and P. Miller. 2021. Treatment disparities among the Black population and their influence on the equitable management of chronic pain. *Health Equity* 5(1):596–605.

Kong, L., J. Ren, S. Fang, T. He, X. Zhou, and M. Fang. 2022. Traditional Chinese exercises on pain and disability in middle-aged and elderly patients with neck pain: A systematic-review and meta-analysis of randomized controlled trials. *Frontiers in Aging Neuroscience* 14:912945.

Kraal, T., I. Sierevelt, D. van Deurzen, M. P. van den Bekerom, and L. Beimers. 2018. Corticosteroid injection alone vs additional physiotherapy treatment in early stage frozen shoulders. *World Journal of Orthopedics* 9(9):165–172. https://doi.org/10.5312/wjo.v9.i9.165.

Lagerbäck, T., G. Kastrati, H. Möller, K. Jensen, M. Skorpil, and P. Gerdhem. 2021. MRI characteristics at a mean of thirteen years after lumbar disc herniation surgery in adolescents: A case-control study. *The Journal of Bone & Joint Surgery* 6(4).

Lanoye, A., K. E. Stewart, B. D. Rybarczyk, S. M. Auerbach, E. Sadock, A. Aggarwal, R. Waller, S. Wolver, and K. Austin. 2017. The impact of integrated psychological services in a safety net primary care clinic on medical utilization. *Journal of Clinical Psychology* 73(6):681–692.

Larkey, L., R. Jahnke, J. Etnier, and J. Gonzalez. 2009. Meditative movement as a category of exercise: Implications for research. *Journal of Physical Activity and Health* 6(2):230–238.

Lauche, R., C. Stumpe, J. Fehr, H. Cramer, Y. W. Cheng, P. M. Wayne, T. Rampp, J. Langhorst, and G. Dobos. 2016. The effects of tai chi and neck exercises in the treatment of chronic nonspecific neck pain: A randomized controlled trial. *The Journal of Pain* 17(9):1013–1027.

Leininger, B., R. Evans, C. M. Greco, L. Hanson, C. Schulz, M. Schneider, J. Connett, F. Keefe, R. M. Glick, and G. Bronfort. 2025. Supported biopsychosocial self-management for back-related leg pain: A randomized feasibility study integrating a whole person perspective. *Chiropractic & Manual Therapies* 33(1):6.

Lybarger, K., M. Yetisgen, and Ö. Uzuner. 2023. The 2022 n2c2/UW shared task on extracting social determinants of health. *Journal of the American Medical Informatics Association* 30(8):1367–1378.

Lyes, M., K. H. Yang, J. Castellanos, and T. Furnish. 2023. Microdosing psilocybin for chronic pain: A case series. *Pain* 164(4):698–702.

Ma, T. W., A. S. Yuen, and Z. Yang. 2023. The efficacy of acceptance and commitment therapy for chronic pain: A systematic review and meta analysis. *The Clinical Journal of Pain* 39(3):147–157.

Mackey, S., H. T. Greely, and K. T. Martucci. 2019. Neuroimaging-based pain biomarkers: Definitions, clinical and research applications, and evaluation frameworks to achieve personalized pain medicine. *PAIN Reports* 4(4):e762.

Mackey, S., N. Aghaeepour, B. Gaudilliere, M. C. Kao, M. Kaptan, E. Lannon, D. Pfyffer, and K. Weber. 2025. Innovations in acute and chronic pain biomarkers: Enhancing diagnosis and personalized therapy. *Regional Anesthesia & Pain Medicine* 50(2):110–120.

MacKichan, F., V. Wylde, and P. Dieppe. 2008. The assessment of musculoskeletal pain in the clinical setting. *Rheumatic Disease Clinics of North America* 34(2):311–330.

Maddox, T., C. Sparks, L. Oldstone, R. Maddox, K. Ffrench, H. Garcia, P. Krishnamurthy, D. Okhotin, L. M. Garcia, B. J. Birckhead, J. Sackman, I. Mackey, R. Louis, V. Salmasi, A. Oyao, and B. D. Darnall. 2023. Durable chronic low back pain reductions up to 24 months after treatment for an accessible, 8-week, in-home behavioral skills-based virtual reality program: A randomized controlled trial. *Pain Medicine* 24(10):1200–1203.

Mahrer, N. E., J. I. Gold, M. Luu, and P. M. Herman. 2018. A cost-analysis of an interdisciplinary pediatric chronic pain clinic. *The Journal of Pain* 19(2):158–165.

Main, C. J., L. A. Ballengee, S. Z. George, J. M. Beneciuk, C. M. Greco, and C. B. Simon. 2023. Psychologically informed practice: The importance of communication in clinical implementation. *Physical Therapy* 103(7).

Maixner, W., R. B. Fillingim, D. A. Williams, S. B. Smith, and G. D. Slade. 2016. Overlapping chronic pain conditions: Implications for diagnosis and classification. *The Journal of Pain* 17(9 Suppl):t93–t107.

Manchikanti, L., V. Pampati, F. J. E. Falco, and J. A. Hirsch. 2015. An updated assessment of utilization of interventional pain management techniques in the Medicare population: 2000-2013. *Pain Physician* 18:E115-E127.

McCracken, L. M., and K. E. Vowles. 2014. Acceptance and commitment therapy and mindfulness for chronic pain: Model, process, and progress. *American Psychologist* 69(2):178–187.

McDonagh, M. S., S. S. Selph, D. I. Buckley, R. S. Holmes, K. Mauer, S. Ramirez, F. C. Hsu, T. Dana, R. Fu, and R. Chou. 2020. Nonopioid pharmacologic treatments for chronic pain. Comparative Effectiveness Review No. 228. (Prepared by the Pacific Northwest Evidence-based Practice Center under Contract No. 290-2015-00009-I.) AHRQ Publication No. 20-EHC010. Rockville, MD: Agency for Healthcare Research and Quality. https://doi.org/10.23970/AHRQEPCCER228.

Meijer, F. S., C. H. Martini, S. Broens, M. Boon, M. Niesters, L. Aarts, E. Olofsen, M. van Velzen, and A. Dahan. 2019. Nociception-guided versus standard care during remifentanil-propofol anesthesia: A randomized controlled trial. *Anesthesiology* 130(5):745–755.

Melek, S. P., D. T. Norris, J. Paulus, K. Matthews, A. Weaver, and S. Davenport. 2018. *Potential economic impact of integrated medical-behavioral healthcare.* Seattle, WA: Millman.

Mezei, L., and B. B. Murinson. 2011. Pain education in North American medical schools. *The Journal of Pain* 12(12):1199–1208.

Morone, N. E., B. L. Rollman, C. G. Moore, Q. Li, and D. K. Weiner. 2009. A mind-body program for older adults with chronic low back pain: Results of a pilot study. *Pain Medicine* 10(8):1395–1407.

Moshrif, A., A. Mosallam, M. H. Abu-Zaid, and W. Gouda. 2023. Evaluating the effect of delayed diagnosis on disease outcome in fibromyalgia: A multi-center cross-sectional study. *Journal of Pain Research* 16:1355–1365.

Murray, C. B., C. B. Groenewald, R. de la Vega, and T. M. Palermo. 2020. Long-term impact of adolescent chronic pain on young adult educational, vocational, and social outcomes. *Pain* 161(2):439–445.

Nahin, R. L., T. Feinberg, F. P. Kapos, and G. W. Terman. 2023. Estimated rates of incident and persistent chronic pain among US adults, 2019–2020. *JAMA Network Open* 6(5):e2313563. https://doi.org/10.1001/jamanetworkopen.2023.13563.

Nahin, R. L., A. Rhee, and B. Stussman. 2024. Use of complementary health approaches overall and for pain management by US adults. *JAMA* 331(7):613–615.

NASEM (National Academies of Sciences, Engineering, and Medicine). 2017. *The health effects of cannabis and cannabinoids: The current state of evidence and recommendations for research.* Washington, DC: The National Academies Press.

National Center for Health Statistics. 2023. NCHS Rapid Surveys System: Round 1 survey description. Hyattsville, MD.

Neville, A., A. Jordan, T. Pincus, C. Nania, F. Schulte, K. O. Yeates, and M. Noel. 2020. Diagnostic uncertainty in pediatric chronic pain: Nature, prevalence, and consequences. *Pain Reports* 5(6):e871.

Osypiuk, K., E. Thompson, and P. M. Wayne. 2018. Can tai chi and qigong postures shape our mood? Toward an embodied cognition framework for mind-body research. *Frontiers in Human Neuroscience* 12:174.

Pain Management Best Practices Inter-Agency Task Force. 2019. *Pain management best practices: Updates, gaps, inconsistencies, and recommendations.* Washington, DC: U.S. Department of Health and Human Services.

Palermo, T. M. 2020. Pain prevention and management must begin in childhood: The key role of psychological interventions. *Pain* 161(Suppl):s114–s121.

Palermo, T. M., A. C. Wilson, M. Peters, A. Lewandowski, and H. Somhegyi. 2009. Randomized controlled trial of an Internet-delivered family cognitive-behavioral therapy intervention for children and adolescents with chronic pain. *Pain* 146(1–2):205–213.

Palermo, T. M., R. de la Vega, C. Murray, E. Law, and C. Zhou. 2020. A digital health psychological intervention (WebMAP Mobile) for children and adolescents with chronic pain: Results of a hybrid effectiveness-implementation stepped-wedge cluster randomized trial. *Pain* 161(12):2763–2774.

Palermo, T. M., G. A. Walco, U. R. Paladhi, K. A. Birnie, G. Crombez, R. de la Vega, C. Eccleston, S. Kashikar-Zuck, and A. L. Stone. 2021. Core outcome set for pediatric chronic pain clinical trials: Results from a Delphi poll and consensus meeting. *Pain* 162(10):2539–2547.

Patel, A. B. U., P. Bibawy, Z. Majeed, W. L. Gan, and G. L. Ackland. 2022. Trans-auricular vagus nerve stimulation to reduce perioperative pain and morbidity: Protocol for a single-blind analyser-masked randomised controlled trial. *BJA Open* 2.

Piette, J. D., S. Newman, S. L. Krein, N. Marinec, J. Chen, D. A. Williams, S. N. Edmond, M. Driscoll, K. M. LaChappelle, R. D. Kerns, M. Maly, H. M. Kim, K. B. Farris, D. M. Higgins, E. Buta, and A. A. Heapy. 2022. Patient-centered pain care using artificial intelligence and mobile health tools: A randomized comparative effectiveness trial. *JAMA Internal Medicine* 182(9):975–983.

Pitcher, M. H., M. Von Korff, M. C. Bushnell, and L. Porter. 2019. Prevalence and profile of high-impact chronic pain in the United States. *The Journal of Pain* 20(2):146–160.

Postier, A. C., D. Eull, C. Schulz, M. Fitzgerald, B. Symalla, D. Watson, L. Goertzen, and S. J. Friedrichsdorf. 2018. Pain experience in a US children's hospital: A point prevalence survey undertaken after the implementation of a system-wide protocol to eliminate or decrease pain caused by needles. *Hospital Pediatrics* 8(9):515–523.

Price, D. D., A. Rafii, L. R. Watkins, and B. Buckingham. 1984. A psychophysical analysis of acupuncture analgesia. *Pain* 19(1):27–42.

Pritzlaff, S. G., U. Latif, J. M. Rosenow, J. Chae, R. D. Wilson, W. J. Huffman, N. D. Crosby, and J. W. Boggs. 2024. A review of prospective studies regarding percutaneous peripheral nerve stimulation treatment in the management of chronic pain. *Pain Management* 14(4):209–222.

Pritzlaff, S. G., N. Singh, C. Sanghvi, M. J. Jung, P. K. Cheng, and D. Copenhaver. 2025. Declining pain medicine fellowship applications from 2019 to 2024: A concerning trend among anesthesia residents and a growing gender disparity. *Pain Practice* 25(1):e13441.

Qaseem, A., T. J. Wilt, R. M. McLean, M. A. Forciea, T. D. Denberg, M. J. Barry, C. Boyd, R. D. Chow, N. Fitterman, R. P. Harris, L. L. Humphrey, and S. Vijan. 2017. Noninvasive treatments for acute, subacute, and chronic low back pain: A clinical practice guideline from the American College of Physicians. *Annals of Internal Medicine* 166(7):514–530.

Rikard, S. M., A. E. Strahan, K. M. Schmit, and G. P. Guy Jr. 2023. Prevalence of pharmacologic and nonpharmacologic pain management therapies among adults with chronic pain—United States, 2020. *Annals of Internal Medicine* 176(11):1571–1575.

Ruehr, L., S. Blomé, G. Kastrati, T. Lagerbäck, M. Jonsjö, H. Möller, M. Skorpil, J. Lasselin, M. Lalouni, P. Gerdhem, and K. Jensen. 2024. Back morphology and walking patterns mean 13.8 years after surgery for lumbar disk herniation in adolescents. *Pain Reports* 9(2):e1148.

Rufener, L., C. Akre, P. Y. Rodondi, and J. Dubois. 2024. Management of chronic non-cancer pain by primary care physicians: A qualitative study. *PLoS One* 19(7):e0307701.

Salaffi, F., S. Farah, B. Bianchi, M. G. Lommano, and M. Di Carlo. 2024. Delay in fibromyalgia diagnosis and its impact on the severity and outcome: A large cohort study. *Clinical and Experimental Rheumatology* 42(6):1198–1204.

Schirle, L., D. C. Samuels, A. Faucon, N. J. Cox, and S. Bruehl. 2023. Polygenic contributions to chronic overlapping pain conditions in a large electronic health record sample. *The Journal of Pain* 24(6):1056–1068.

Schmalzl, L., and C. E. Kerr. 2016. Editorial: Neural mechanisms underlying movement-based embodied contemplative practices. *Frontiers in Human Neuroscience* 10.

Schrepf, A., W. Maixner, R. Fillingim, C. Veasley, R. Ohrbach, S. Smith, and D. A. Williams. 2024. The chronic overlapping pain condition screener. *The Journal of Pain* 25(1):265–272.

Simons, L. E., C. B. Sieberg, M. Pielech, C. Conroy, and D. E. Logan. 2013. What does it take? Comparing intensive rehabilitation to outpatient treatment for children with significant pain-related disability. *Journal of Pediatric Psychology* 38(2):213–223.

Simons, L. E., A. Smith, C. Ibagon, R. Coakley, D. E. Logan, N. Schechter, D. Borsook, and J. C. Hill. 2015. Pediatric Pain Screening Tool: Rapid identification of risk in youth with pain complaints. *Pain* 156(8):1511–1518.

Simons, L. E., C. B. Sieberg, C. Conroy, E. T. Randall, J. Shulman, D. Borsook, C. Berde, N. F. Sethna, and D. E. Logan. 2018. Children with chronic pain: Response trajectories following intensive pain rehabilitation treatment. *The Journal of Pain* 19(2):207–218.

Simons, L. E., J. W. S. Vlaeyen, L. Declercq, A. M. Smith, J. Beebe, M. Hogan, E. Li, C. A. Kronman, F. Mahmud, J. R. Corey, C. B. Sieberg, and C. Ploski. 2020. Avoid or engage? Outcomes of graded exposure in youth with chronic pain using a sequential replicated single-case randomized design. *Pain* 161(3):520–531. https://doi.org/10.1097/j.pain.0000000000001735.

Simons, L. E., L. E. Harrison, D. B. Boothroyd, G. Parvathinathan, A. R. Van Orden, S. F. O'Brien, D. Schofield, J. Kraindler, R. Shrestha, J. W. S. Vlaeyen, and R. K. Wicksell. 2024. A randomized controlled trial of graded exposure treatment (GET living) for adolescents with chronic pain. *Pain* 165(1):177–191.

Skelly, A. C., R. Chou, J. R. Dettori, J. A. Turner, J. L. Friedly, S. D. Rundell, R. Fu, E. D. Brodt, N. Wasson, S. Kantner, and A. J. R. Ferguson. 2020. Noninvasive nonpharmacological treatment for chronic pain: A systematic review update. AHRQ Comparative Effectiveness Reviews. Report No. 20-EHC009. Rockville, MD: Agency for Healthcare Research and Quality.

Stenum, J., M. M. Hsu, A. Y. Pantelyat, and R. T. Roemmich. 2024. Clinical gait analysis using video-based pose estimation: Multiple perspectives, clinical populations, and measuring change. *PLOS Digital Health* 3(3):e0000467.

Stone, A. L., A. L. Holley, N. F. Dieckmann, and A. C. Wilson. 2019. Use of the PROMIS-29® to identify subgroups of mothers with chronic pain. *Health Psychology* 38(5):422–430.

Tan, G., D. H. Rintala, M. P. Jensen, J. S. Richards, S. A. Holmes, R. Parachuri, S. Lashgari-Saegh, and L. R. Price. 2011. Efficacy of cranial electrotherapy stimulation for neuropathic pain following spinal cord injury: A multi-site randomized controlled trial with a secondary 6-month open-label phase. *The Journal of Spinal Cord Medicine* 34(3):285–296.

Tang, L., Z. Sun, B. Idnay, J. G. Nestor, A. Soroush, P. A. Elias, Z. Xu, Y. Ding, G. Durrett, J. F. Rousseau, C. Weng, and Y. Peng. 2023. Evaluating large language models on medical evidence summarization. *NPJ Digital Med* 6(1):158.

Taylor, K. A., F. P. Kapos, J. A. Sharpe, A. S. Kosinski, D. I. Rhon, and A. P. Goode. 2024. Seventeen-year national pain prevalence trends among U.S. military veterans. *The Journal of Pain* 25(5):104420.

Tiecke, E., M. Rainisio, E. Eisenberg, J. Wainstein, E. Kaplan, M. Silverberg, L. Hochman, and S. Mangialaio. 2022. NRD.E1, an innovative non-opioid therapy for painful diabetic peripheral neuropathy—A randomized proof of concept study. *European Journal of Pain* 26(8):1665–1678.

Tracy, I., and P. W. Mantyh. 2007. The cerebral signature for pain perception and its modulation. *Neuron* (55)3. https://doi.org/10.1016/j.neuron.2007.07.012.

U.S. Department of Health and Human Services. 2019. *Pain management best practices interagency task force report: Updates, gaps, inconsistencies, and recommendations.* https://www.hhs.gov/sites/default/files/pain-mgmt-best-practices-draft-final-report-05062019.pdf (accessed May 13, 2025).

U.S. Food and Drug Administration. 2018. Methods to identify what is important to patients & select, develop or modify fit-for-purpose clinical outcomes assessments. https://www.fda.gov/media/116277/download (accessed July 15, 2025).

Van Veen, D., C. Van Uden, L. Blankemeier, J. B. Delbrouck, A. Aali, C. Bluethgen, A. Pareek, M. Polacin, E. P. Reis, A. Seehofnerová, N. Rohatgi, P. Hosamani, W. Collins, N. Ahuja, C. P. Langlotz, J. Hom, S. Gatidis, J. Pauly, and A. S. Chaudhari. 2024. Adapted large language models can outperform medical experts in clinical text summarization. *Nature Medicine* 30(4):1134–1142.

Vaughn, I. A., E. L. Terry, E. J. Bartley, N. Schaefer, and R. B. Fillingim. 2019. Racial-ethnic differences in osteoarthritis pain and disability: A meta-analysis. *The Journal of Pain* 20(6):629–644.

Vickers, A. J., A. M. Cronin, A. C. Maschino, G. Lewith, H. MacPherson, N. E. Foster, K. J. Sherman, C. M. Witt, and K. Linde. 2012. Acupuncture for chronic pain: Individual patient data meta-analysis. *JAMA Internal Medicine* 172(19):1444–1453.

Von Korff, M., L. L. DeBar, E. E. Krebs, R. D. Kerns, R. A. Deyo, and F. J. Keefe. 2020. Graded chronic pain scale revised: Mild, bothersome, and high-impact chronic pain. *Pain* 161(3):651–661.

Voss, S., D. A. Boachie, N. Nieves, and N. P. Gothe. 2023. Mind-body practices, interoception and pain: A scoping review of behavioral and neural correlates. *Annals of Medicine* 55(2):2275661.

Vydiswaran, V. G. V., A. Strayhorn, K. Weber, H. Stevens, J. Mellinger, G. S. Winder, and A. C. Fernandez. 2024. Automated-detection of risky alcohol use prior to surgery using natural language processing. *Alcoholism: Clinical and Experimental Research* 48(1):153–163.

Wakefield, E. O., V. Belamkar, M. D. Litt, R. M. Puhl, and W. T. Zempsky. 2022. "There's nothing wrong with you": Pain-related stigma in adolescents with chronic pain. *Journal of Pediatric Psychology* 47(4):456–468.

Walker, L. S., A. L. Stone, G. T. Han, J. Garber, S. Bruehl, C. A. Smith, J. Anderson, and T. M. Palermo. 2021. Internet-delivered cognitive behavioral therapy for youth with functional abdominal pain: A randomized clinical trial testing differential efficacy by patient subgroup. *Pain* 162(12):2945–2955.

Wang, C., C. H. Schmid, M. D. Iversen, W. F. Harvey, R. A. Fielding, J. B. Driban, L. L. Price, J. B. Wong, K. F. Reid, R. Rones, and T. McAlindon. 2016. Comparative effectiveness of tai chi versus physical therapy for knee osteoarthritis: A randomized trial. *Annals of Internal Medicine* 165(2):77–86.

Wayne, P., and M. Fuerst. 2013. *The Harvard Medical School guide to tai chi: 12 weeks to a healthy body, strong heart, and sharp mind.* Boston: Shambhala.

Wilson, R. D., D. D. Gunzler, M. E. Bennett, and J. Chae. 2014. Peripheral nerve stimulation compared with usual care for pain relief of hemiplegic shoulder pain: A randomized controlled trial. *American Journal of Physical Medicine &Rehabilitation* 93(1):17–28.

Wood, L., N. E. Foster, S. G. Dean, V. Booth, J. A. Hayden, and A. Booth. 2024. Contexts, behavioural mechanisms and outcomes to optimise therapeutic exercise prescription for persistent low back pain: A realist review. *British Journal of Sports Medicine* 58(4):222–230.

Woods, S. B., P. N. E. Roberson, Q. Booker, B. L. Wood, and S. Q. Booker. 2024. Longitudinal associations of family relationship quality with chronic pain incidence and persistence among aging African Americans. *The Journals of Gerontology. Series B, Psychological Sciences and Social Sciences* 79(7).

Yang, G. Y., J. Hunter, F. L. Bu, W. L. Hao, H. Zhang, P. M. Wayne, and J. P. Liu. 2022. Determining the safety and effectiveness of tai chi: A critical overview of 210 systematic reviews of controlled clinical trials. *Systematic Review* 11(1):260.

Yang, Y., S. McCluskey, M. Bydon, J. R. Singh, R. D. Sheeler, K. R. Nathani, A. C. Krieger, N. D. Mehta, J. Weaver, L. Jia, S. DeCelle, R. C. Schlagal, J. Ayar, S. Abduljawad, S. D. Stovitz, R. Ganesh, J. Verkuilen, K. A. Knapp, L. Yang, and R. Härtl. 2024. A tai chi and qigong mind-body program for low back pain: A virtually delivered randomized control trial. *North American Spine Society* 20:100557.

Zeliadt, S. B., E. R. Thomas, J. Olson, S. Coggeshall, K. Giannitrapani, P. E. Ackland, K. P. Reddy, D. G. Federman, D. F. Drake, B. Kligler, and S. L. Taylor. 2020. Patient feedback on the effectiveness of auricular acupuncture on pain in routine clinical care: The experience of 11,406 veterans. *MedCare* 58 (29 Suppl):s101–s107.

Ziadni, M. S., S. R. Anderson, L. Gonzalez-Castro, and B. D. Darnall. 2021. Efficacy of a single-session "empowered relief" zoom-delivered group intervention for chronic pain: Randomized controlled trial conducted during the COVID-19 pandemic. *Journal of Medical Internet Research* 23(9):e29672. https://doi.org/10.2196/29672.

Zick, S. M., A. Sen, G. K. Wyatt, S. L. Murphy, J. T. Arnedt, and R. E. Harris. 2016. Investigation of 2 types of self-administered acupressure for persistent cancer-related fatigue in breast cancer survivors: A randomized clinical trial. *JAMA Oncology* 2(11):1470–1476.

Appendix A

Workshop Agenda

DAY 1: THURSDAY, APRIL 17, 2025

Purpose
- Discuss how the wide variety of experiences and challenges related to chronic pain and its management impact an individual's health status, functional limitations, and medical records for children and adults.
- Consider best practices and methods of categorization for chronic pain and advancements in the treatment, management, and measurement of individuals' chronic pain levels for children and adults.
- Highlight special considerations in how medical providers approach treatment of different severities in chronic pain for children and adults.
- Explore alternative and complementary pain treatments pursued by individuals experiencing chronic pain, the efficacy of those treatments, how they may be reflected in the medical record, and implications for, or interactions with, traditional treatment paradigms.
- Consider the lived experiences of people with chronic pain as they seek medical care and navigate the Social Security Administration (SSA) disability system.
- Receive an overview of recent or emerging research on new or improved methods for the measurement and management of chronic pain.

9:00 am   **Welcome and Overview of Workshop**
Allen Heinemann, Northwestern University Feinberg School of Medicine and Shirley Ryan AbilityLab, *Planning Committee Chair*

9:05 am   **Sponsor Remarks & Overview of SSA Disability Evaluation Policy**
Robert Weathers, Social Security Administration
Vincent Nibali, Social Security Administration

9:30 am   **General Overview, Concepts, and Framing of Chronic Pain and Disability**
Moderator: Allen Heinemann, Northwestern University Feinberg School of Medicine and Shirley Ryan AbilityLab, *Planning Committee Chair*

Clinical and Patient Experiences of Chronic Pain
Kim Dupree Jones, Emory University, *Planning Committee Member*
Legal and Regulatory Conceptions of Chronic Pain
Jerome Bickenbach, University of Lucerne (virtual)

9:50 am   **Audience Q&A**

10:00 am   **Session 1: Factors Affecting Access to Effective Chronic Pain Care**
Moderator: Tamara Baker, University of North Carolina at Chapel Hill, *Planning Committee Member*
Objectives:
- Consider the lived experiences of people with chronic pain as they seek medical care and navigate the SSA disability system.
- Discuss how the wide variety of experiences and challenges related to chronic pain and its management impact an individual's health status, functional limitations, and medical records for children and adults.
- Explore how variations in access to chronic pain interventions can impact the care that individuals receive and the health outcomes they experience.

10:00 am   **Speaker Presentations**
Jaime Sanders, individual with migraine lived experience
Edwin Aroke, University of Alabama
Staja Booker, University of Florida (virtual)

10:35 am   **Moderated Panel and Audience Q&A**
Tamara Baker, University of North Carolina at Chapel Hill,
    Planning Committee Member

11:00 am   **BREAK**

11:15 am   **Session 2: Methods and Metrics for Chronic Pain Assessment in Adults and Children**
Moderator: Reuben Escorpizo, University of Vermont,
    Planning Committee Member
Objectives:
- Consider the lived experiences of people with chronic pain as they seek medical care and navigate the SSA disability system.
- Consider best practices and methods of categorization for chronic pain and advancements in the treatment, management, and measurement of individuals' chronic pain levels for children and adults.
- Discuss how the assessment of chronic pain connects to assessments of function, performance, behavior, and disability.

11:15 am   **Speaker Presentations**
Deb Constien, individual with chronic pain lived experience
Steven George, Duke University
Carole A. Tucker, University of Texas Medical Branch
Anna Wilson, Oregon Health & Science University

12:05 pm   **Moderated Panel and Audience Q&A**
Reuben Escorpizo, University of Vermont, *Planning Committee Member*

12:30 pm   **LUNCH**

1:30 pm   **Session 3: Best Practices and Clinician Perspectives on Chronic Pain Treatment and Management in Children**
Moderator: Henry Xiang, The Ohio State University School of Medicine and Nationwide Children's Hospital, *Planning Committee Member*
Objectives:
- Consider the lived experiences of people with chronic pain as they seek medical care and navigate the SSA disability system.
- Consider best practices and methods of categorization for chronic pain and advancements in the treatment, management, and measurement of individuals' chronic pain levels for children.
- Highlight special considerations in how medical providers approach treatment of different severities in chronic pain for children.

1:30 pm   **Speaker Presentations**
Casey Cashman, U.S. Pain Foundation
Tonya Palermo, Seattle Children's Hospital (virtual)
Stefan Friedrichsdorf, University of California, San Francisco (virtual)
Laura Simons, Stanford University

2:15 pm   **Moderated Panel and Audience Q&A**
Henry Xiang, The Ohio State University School of Medicine and Nationwide Children's Hospital, *Planning Committee Member*

2:40 pm   **BREAK**

2:50 pm   **Session 4: Best Practices on Chronic Pain Treatment and Management in Adults**
Moderator: Christopher Standaert, University of Pittsburgh, *Planning Committee Member*
Objectives:
- Describe best practices and methods of categorization for chronic pain and advancements in the treatment, management, and measurement of individuals' chronic pain levels for adults.
- Discuss the degree to which various types of chronic pain treatments alleviate functional limitations.

2:50 pm	**Speaker Presentations** Kemly Philip, University of Texas Medical Center Carol Greco, University of Pittsburgh Julie Fritz, University of Utah
3:20 pm	**Moderated Panel and Audience Q&A** Christopher Standaert, University of Pittsburgh, *Planning Committee Member*
3:45 pm	**BREAK**
3:55 pm	**Session 5: Patient Journeys and Clinician Perspectives in Treatment and Management of Chronic Pain** Moderator: Juan Hincapie-Castillo, University of North Carolina at Chapel Hill, *Planning Committee Member* Objectives: • Discuss the lived experiences of people with chronic pain as they seek medical care and navigate the SSA disability system. • Highlight special considerations in how medical providers approach treatment of different severities in chronic pain for adults. • Describe challenges in continuity of care for people living with chronic pain.
3:55 pm	**Speaker Presentations** Anna Williams, Clusterbusters, *Planning Committee Member* Joseph Cammilleri, University of Florida, Jacksonville Shravani Durbhakula, Vanderbilt School of Medicine
4:25 pm	**Moderated Panel and Audience Q&A** Juan Hincapie-Castillo, University of North Carolina at Chapel Hill, *Planning Committee Member*
4:50 pm	**Closing Remarks** Allen Heinemann, Northwestern University Feinberg School of Medicine and Shirley Ryan AbilityLab, *Planning Committee Chair*
5:00 pm	**END OF DAY 1**

DAY 2: FRIDAY, APRIL 18, 2025

9:00 am   **Recap of Day 1 and Plans for Day 2**
Allen Heinemann, Northwestern University School of Medicine and Shirley Ryan AbilityLab, *Planning Committee Chair*

9:05 am   **Session 6: Health Care System Challenges in Comprehensive Chronic Pain Management**
Moderator: Kim Dupree Jones, Emory University, *Planning Committee Member*
Objectives:
- Consider the lived experiences of people with chronic pain as they seek medical care and navigate the SSA disability system.
- Discuss how the wide variety of experiences and challenges related to chronic pain and its management impact an individual's health status, functional limitations, and medical records for children and adults.
- Explore systemic barriers to delivering comprehensive, evidence-based pain care across various health care settings, including federally qualified health centers (FQHCs), primary care practices, and academic health centers.

9:05 am   **Speaker Presentations**
Andrea Anderson, individual with chronic pain lived experience (virtual)
Beth Darnall, Stanford University
Julie Fritz, University of Utah
V. G. Vinod Vydiswaran, University of Michigan

9:50 am   **Moderated Panel and Audience Q&A**
Kim Dupree Jones, Emory University, *Planning Committee Member*

10:15 am   **Session 7: Complementary and Alternative Therapies in Comprehensive Chronic Pain Management**
Moderator: Kim Dupree Jones, Emory University, *Planning Committee Member*
Objectives:
- Consider the lived experiences of people with chronic pain as they seek medical care and navigate the SSA disability system.

> - Explore alternative and complementary pain treatments pursued by individuals experiencing chronic pain, the efficacy of those treatments, how they may be reflected in the medical record, and implications for, or interactions with, traditional treatment paradigms.
> - Explore the integration of complementary and alternative medicine into conventional pain care to enhance physical, social, and psychological outcomes.

10:15 am   **Speaker Presentations**
Tom Norris, American Chronic Pain Association (virtual)
Peter Wayne, Harvard Medical School
Richard Harris, University of California, Irvine (virtual)
Anna Woodbury, Emory University

10:50 am   **Moderated Panel and Audience Q&A**
Kim Dupree Jones, Emory University, *Planning Committee Member*

11:15 am   **BREAK**

11:30 am   **Session 8: Emerging Research on New or Improved Methods for the Measurement and Management of Chronic Pain**
Moderator: Sean Mackey, Stanford University, *Planning Committee Member*
Objective:
- Receive an overview of recent or emerging research on new or improved methods for the measurement and management of chronic pain.

11:30 am   **Speaker Presentations**
Sean Mackey, Stanford University, *Planning Committee Member*
Nat Schuster, University of California, San Diego (virtual)
Konstantin Slavin, University of Illinois
John Chae, Case Western Reserve University
Ming Jeffrey Kao, Stanford University (virtual)
Christin Veasley, Chronic Pain Research Alliance (virtual)

12:30 pm   **Moderated Panel and Audience Q&A**
Sean Mackey, Stanford University, *Planning Committee Member*

1:00 pm   **Session 9: Key Challenges and Opportunities in Chronic Pain and Disability**
Moderator: Allen Heinemann, Northwestern University Feinberg School of Medicine and Shirley Ryan AbilityLab, *Planning Committee Chair*
Objective:
- Highlight key themes discussed throughout the workshop.

Planning Committee Members
Tamara Baker, University of North Carolina at Chapel Hill
Reuben Escorpizo, University of Vermont
Henry Xiang, The Ohio State University and Nationwide Children's Hospital
Christopher Standaert, University of Pittsburgh
Anna Williams, Clusterbusters
Juan Hincapie-Castillo, University of North Carolina at Chapel Hill
Kim Dupree Jones, Emory University
Sean Mackey, Stanford University
Anirban Basu, University of Washington (virtual)

1:25 pm   **Closing Remarks**
Allen Heinemann, Northwestern University Feinberg School of Medicine and Shirley Ryan AbilityLab, *Planning Committee Chair*

1:30 pm   **MEETING ADJOURNS**

Appendix B

Biographical Sketches of the Planning Committee and Workshop Speakers

Andrea Anderson has served as a national advocate for people living with persistent and high-impact pain since 2017. Today, her primary focus is collaborating with researchers and academic institutions to advance research, prevention, and potential cures for chronic and severe pain. She is involved in projects with several leading universities, including the University of Houston, Stanford University, the University of Michigan, and the University of Texas. Her work centers on bridging the gap between academia and patients—ensuring patient experiences are prioritized and helping connect individuals with relevant research opportunities. Her work includes partnerships with the Food and Drug Administration; Centers for Medicare & Medicaid Services; National Institutes of Health; Centers for Disease Control and Prevention; National Academies of Sciences, Engineering, and Medicine; the Bree Collaborative; and the American Academy of Hospice and Palliative Medicine. She has played a key role in advocating for and developing both state and federal legislation and has testified at state medical board hearings on behalf of chronic pain patients. She serves as an adviser to the National Pain Advocacy Center and was the executive director of the Alliance for the Treatment of Intractable Pain. In addition to her advocacy work, Anderson is a legal consultant for medical malpractice and personal injury cases.

Edwin Aroke, PhD, CRNA, is an internationally recognized CRNA scientist who specializes in pain research and health disparities. He is a tenured associate professor and the assistant dean for research and scholarship at the University of Alabama at Birmingham School of Nursing. Aroke's

National Institutes of Health–funded research program examines the role of epigenomic changes in chronic pain and pain disparities. His international leadership seeks to enhance equity in anesthesia outcomes. Aroke cofounded the Association of Cameroonian Nurse Anesthetists in America, and as association president he led initiatives to improve anesthesia outcomes in Cameroon. Among his numerous awards are the Researcher of the Year from the American Association of Nurse Anesthesiology Foundation and the Founders Award for Excellence in Genomic Nursing Research from the International Society of Nurses in Genetics. Aroke is a fellow of the Academy of Diversity Leaders in Nursing, the American Association of Nurse Anesthesiology, and the American Academy of Nursing.

Tamara Baker, PhD, MA, (Planning Committee Member) is a professor in the Department of Psychiatry at the University of North Carolina at Chapel Hill. She is an appointed member of the U.S. Department of Veterans Affairs Geriatric and Gerontology Advisory Committee and a member of the National Institutes of Health's Interagency Pain Research Coordinating Committee. She is the editor in chief of *Ethnicity & Health*, and has served as the former secretary and chair of the Committee on Minority Issues in Gerontology, and chair of the Behavioral and Social Sciences section for the Gerontological Society of America (GSA). She is a GSA Fellow, founder and co-convener of GSA's Historically Black Colleges and Universities Collaborative Interest Group, and GSA Board of Governor's Vice President Elect. Her background in gerontology, psychology, and biobehavioral health has evolved into an active research agenda that focuses on understanding the behavioral and psychosocial predictors and outcomes of chronic pain and pain and symptom management among older adults from historically marginalized populations. More broadly, her research includes health disparities and health equity, cultural diversity and sensitivity, and social determinants of health. Dr. Baker received her PhD from Penn State University and MA from Norfolk State University.

Anirban Basu, PhD, MS, (Planning Committee Member) is a professor of health economics and the Stergachis Family Endowed Director of the CHOICE Institute at the University of Washington, Seattle, with joint appointments in the Departments of Health Systems & Population Health and Economics. He is a research associate at the U.S. National Bureau of Economic Research and an elected fellow at the American Statistical Association. His research focuses on understanding the economic value of health care, generating causal evidence, and understanding the potential for discrimination with machine learning and artificial intelligence algorithms. From 2018 to 2024, he co-led the National Heart, Lung, and Blood Institute's Cure Sickle Cell Consortium on Economic Impact and Analysis.

He served on the 2nd Panel on Cost-effectiveness Analysis in Health and Medicine and serves on the editorial advisory board for *Value in Health* journal. Basu has earned many academic honors, including the 2018 Mid-Career Excellence Award from the Health Policy Statistics Section of the American Statistical Association, the 2007 and 2016 Research Excellence Award for Methodological Excellence, and the 2009 Bernie O'Brien New Investigator Award from the International Society for Pharmacoeconomics and Outcomes Research. He received his MS in biostatistics from the University of North Carolina at Chapel Hill and a PhD in public policy studies from the University of Chicago.

Jerome Bickenbach, PhD, LLB, is permanent visiting professor at the University of Lucerne and professor emeritus at Queen's University, Canada. He is the author or editor of several books on disability law and policy. As a consultant to World Health Organization, Bickenbach worked on developing and finalizing the International Classification of Functioning, Disability and Health, and more recently on the Rehabilitation 2030 initiative, and as consultant with the World Bank, United Nations Children's Fund, and the Organisation for Economic Co-operation and Development has assisted several countries in reforming disability assessment and disability needs assessment tools. His research spans various aspects of disability studies, including quality of life of persons with disability, disability epidemiology, participatory action, inclusion, modeling disability statistics for population health surveys, the relationship between disability and health, and the ethics and the application of International Classification of Functioning, Disability and Health to monitoring the implementation of the United Nations Convention on the Rights of Persons with Disabilities. As a lawyer in Canada, Bickenbach was a human rights litigator, specializing in anti-discrimination for persons with intellectual impairments and mental illness.

Staja "Star" Booker, PhD, is an assistant professor at the University of Florida College of Nursing. Booker is well known for her research on disparities, injustices, and health equity in the field of pain. For more than 10 years, her research has illuminated the lived experience and management of chronic pain in older adults, specifically those who identify as African American/Black. She has completed several research projects funded by the National Institutes of Health, and her current funded study will test a pain self-management intervention that addresses social determinants of chronic pain. Booker is a fellow of the American Academy of Nursing. She has published nearly 100 peer-reviewed articles and editorials and 9 book chapters and has given more than 130 scientific presentations. In 2022 she was one of 10 faculty from across the University of Florida who received the Excellence Award for Assistant Professors, the first time a College of

Nursing faculty has received this award. Other awards include the Southern Nursing Research Society's Early Science Investigator Award, the International Association for the Study of Pain's Pain in Older Persons Junior Investigator Award, and the American Society of Pain Management Nursing Excellence in Nursing Award for Pain Management of the Older Adult. Booker is an active member and leader in several pain, gerontology, and nursing organizations.

Joseph Cammilleri, PharmD, BCACP, CPE, earned his Doctor of Pharmacy degree from Palm Beach Atlantic University and furthered his clinical expertise through a postgraduate residency at Shands Hospital in Jacksonville, Florida. He enhanced his professional credentials by obtaining board certification in ambulatory care pharmacy in 2012 and completing specialized training through the American Society of Health-System Pharmacists Foundation's pain management and palliative care traineeship program in 2014. In his current role at University of Florida Health Jacksonville, Cammilleri serves as both an ambulatory care clinical pharmacist and program director for the Postgraduate Year Two pain and palliative care residency program. His professional focus centers on pain management and overdose prevention strategies.

Casey Cashman uses her voice to fight passionately for the rights of people with pain, especially children. She has lived most of her life with multiple serious health conditions, including complex regional pain syndrome, postural orthostatic tachycardia syndrome, and Ehlers-Danlos syndrome. Before joining the U.S. Pain Foundation, Cashman spent many years working in human resources. She brings this knowledge and experience to the table in her role as director of the Pediatric Pain Warriors Program, where she provides compassionate support to kids with pain and their families as they travel along their pain journeys. Cashman also spearheads U.S. Pain's fundraising efforts and has helped create various programs and collaborations designed to support the organization's free programs and services.

John Chae, MD, serves as executive vice president and chief academic officer for the MetroHealth System. He serves as senior associate dean for medical affairs and is professor of physical medicine and rehabilitation (PM&R) and biomedical engineering (BME) at the Case Western Reserve University (CWRU) School of Medicine. He served as chair of PM&R at MetroHealth System and CWRU from 2013 to 2023. Chae received his bachelor of science from Duke University and his master's in BME from Dartmouth College. He received his MD from Rutgers University–New Jersey Medical School (NJMS) and his clinical training in PM&R from Rutgers–NJMS and the Kessler Institute for Rehabilitation. He completed the National Institutes of Health Rehabilitation Medicine Scientist Training Program Fellowship at CWRU. Chae is member of the National Academy of Medicine. Chae served as president of the Association of Academic Physiatrists from 2017 to 2019 and received the association's Distinguished Academician Award in 2022. Chae's research focuses on the application of electrical stimulation for neuroprostheses, neural plasticity, and the treatment of musculoskeletal pain. His research team developed percutaneous peripheral nerve stimulation for the treatment of chronic musculoskeletal pain, which is now commercially available and has been placed in more than 32,000 patients. He also co-invented contralaterally controlled functional electrical stimulation for post-stroke motor relearning, which has been transferred to an industry partner and is in the process of commercialization. Chae has more than 135 peer-reviewed publications, books, and book chapters and has been awarded 33 patents.

Deb Constien lives in Sun Prairie, Wisconsin. She was diagnosed with rheumatoid arthritis at the age of 13. She is a medically retired registered dietitian with majors in dietetics and biology. Constien has volunteered for the International Foundation for Autoimmune & Autoinflammatory Arthritis for more than 10 years. She cohosts its podcasts and attends American College of Radiology and European Alliance of Associations for Rheumatology conferences yearly. She has been on the Advisory Council for the Wisconsin Research and Education Network for the past eight years. At the Arthritis Foundation, Constien serves as the cochair of the executive National Advocacy Committee. She has spoken at several press conferences and testified in Congress. Constien also serves as a consumer reviewer for the Department of Defense Congressionally Directed Medical Research Programs.

Beth Darnall, PhD, is professor of anesthesiology, perioperative, and pain medicine at Stanford University Medical School and director of the Stanford Pain Relief Innovations Lab. A psychologist-scientist, she leads National Institutes of Health (NIH) and Patient-Centered Outcomes Research Institute-funded national studies on scalable behavioral analgesic interventions and patient-centered opioid reduction. Her work centers on developing, investigating, and disseminating solutions that offer more equitable access to evidence-based behavioral pain care for diverse and underserved populations. She created Empowered Relief®, a single-session group intervention that rapidly equips individuals with effective pain relief skills for acute, chronic, and postsurgical pain. Empowered Relief® is delivered by certified instructors in 30 countries and in 8 languages. She has three times briefed the U.S. Congress and the Food and Drug Administration on patient-centered pain care and opioid stewardship. She is a scientific member of the NIH Interagency Pain Research Coordinating Committee, served on the Centers for Disease Control and Prevention Opioid Workgroup (2021), is chief science advisor for AppliedVR, and is author of four books for patients and clinicians. She has keynoted national pain society conferences in Australia, New Zealand, the Netherlands, Switzerland, and the UK. In 2018 she spoke on the psychology of pain relief at the World Economic Forum in Davos, Switzerland.

Shravani Durbhakula, MD, MPH, MBA, is a double-board-certified interventional pain physician and anesthesiologist known for her expertise in personalized pain management and education. She has a track record of creating innovative educational products and technological tools to address gaps in pain education and public health outcomes. Her current research focuses on using artificial intelligence to advance precision medicine and optimize therapy utilization in chronic pain. Durbhakula has received numerous accolades, including the 2025 American Society of Regional Anesthesia and Pain Medicine Excellence in Education Award and the 2023 American Academy of Pain Medicine Presidential Excellence Award for Education. She was featured by NPR for her educational innovations, and her research is published in top-tier journals. She serves on the board of directors for the American Academy of Pain Medicine Foundation and hosts the American Academy of Pain Medicine podcast *Pain Matters*. Durbhakula taught at Johns Hopkins School of Medicine, where she directed the first pain curriculum for first-year medical students and the Multidisciplinary Pain Fellowship. Currently at Vanderbilt University School of Medicine, she specializes in treating peripheral nerve injuries and serves on the Vanderbilt University Medical Center's Controlled Substances Quality Oversight Committee and the Executive Admissions Committee for the School of Medicine.

Reuben Escorpizo, PT, MSc, DPT, (Planning Committee Member) is a rehabilitation clinician scientist and academic with established work in the International Classification of Functioning, Disability and Health (ICF) and disability outcomes. He co-led the development of the Clinical Practice Guideline for Physical Therapists in Work Rehabilitation through the American Physical Therapy Association and the Academy of Orthopedic Physical Therapy. He has published 1 book, 22 book chapters/e-chapters, and more than 130 publications, and has numerous invited keynotes and visiting professorships. He has been invited to participate in international work like the ICF-Pain Task Force of the International Association for the Study of Pain, the International Spinal Cord Injury Community Study, the ISCOS Core Data Set Committee for Vocational Rehabilitation, and the Outcome Measures in Rheumatology Worker Productivity group. Dr.

Escorpizo was appointed as the inaugural section chief editor of "Disability, Rehabilitation, and Inclusion" of the journal *Frontiers in Rehabilitation Sciences*. He co-developed the Work Rehabilitation Questionnaire (WORQ), a questionnaire used in rehabilitation settings and translated into multiple languages worldwide. He completed his master's degree in kinesiology (occupational biomechanics), Doctor of Physical Therapy degree, and post-clinical doctorate degree in disability evaluation and rehabilitation. He practices in a general outpatient clinic of the University of Vermont Medical Center and sees diverse patients including those referred for work rehabilitation. He currently serves on the National Academies of Sciences, Engineering, and Medicine Standing Committee of Medical and Vocational Experts for the Social Security Administration's Disability Programs.

Stefan Friedrichsdorf, MD, is a pediatric pain and palliative medicine specialist who treats children experiencing acute and chronic pain. He also provides holistic care for pediatric patients with life-limiting diseases and with his team adds an extra layer of support to the care of children with serious illness and their families. He serves as medical director of the Stad Center for Pediatric Pain, Palliative and Integrative Medicine at Benioff Children's Hospitals in Oakland and San Francisco.

Julie Fritz, PhD, PT, ATC, is a distinguished professor in the Department of Physical Therapy and Athletic Training at the University of Utah. Fritz's research career has focused on developing and evaluating nonpharmacologic interventions for patients with chronic pain. She is a principal investigator for clinical trials investigating nonpharmacologic interventions for persons with chronic musculoskeletal pain funded through the National Institutes of Health–Department of Veterans Affairs–Department of Defense Pain Management Collaboratory, the National Institutes of Health Helping End Long Term Addiction (HEAL) Pragmatic and Implementation Studies for the Management of Pain to Reduce Opioid Prescribing (PRISM) and Back Pain Consortium (BACPAC) programs, Patient-Centered Outcomes Research Institute, and the Department of Defense. Federal agencies have continuously funded Fritz's research since 2008, and her work has included rigorous clinical trials published in high-impact journals. In addition, these studies have provided Fritz with the opportunity to engage with interdisciplinary teams of physical therapists, physicians, behavioral health specialists, informaticists, biostatisticians, and health care economists.

Steven George, PhD, PT, FAPTA, conducts research involving biopsychosocial models for the prevention and treatment of chronic musculoskeletal pain disorders. His long-term goals are to improve accuracy for predicting who is going to develop chronic pain, and to identify nonpharmacological treatment options that limit the development of chronic pain conditions. George is an active member of the American Physical Therapy Association, American Pain Society, and International Association for the Study of Pain. George's research projects have been supported by the National Institutes of Health, Department of Defense, Patient-Centered Outcomes Research Institute, Brooks Rehabilitation, Orthopaedic Section of the American Physical Therapy Association, University of Florida, and Foundation for Physical Therapy. George and his collaborators have authored more than 200 peer-reviewed publications in leading physical therapy, rehabilitation, and pain research journals. He currently serves as a contributing editor for *Physical Therapy* and editorial board member for the *Journal of Pain*. George is also a member of the advisory council for the National Center for Complementary and Integrative Health.

Carol Greco, PhD, is an associate professor in the Department of Psychiatry and the Department of Physical Therapy at the University of Pittsburgh. She is a licensed clinical psychologist and researcher specializing in psychosocial assessment, Patient-Reported Outcomes Measurement Information System (PROMIS) instrument development, and nonpharmacologic interventions such as cognitive behavioral therapy and mindfulness meditation for pain and chronic illness symptoms. She has been principal investigator, site principal investigator, co-investigator, and interventionist on numerous grants and awards from the National Institutes of Health, Patient-Centered Outcomes Research Institute, and foundations. Greco and her team have used PROMIS instrument development methodology to create patient-reported measures of context factors that can affect treatment outcomes, like positive outlook and treatment expectations. Greco has been a co-investigator and trainer on several federally funded research trials designed to reduce the burden of back pain by teaching physical therapists, chiropractors, and other professionals how to implement effective communication and behavioral pain management strategies with their patients.

Richard Harris, PhD, is a Susan Samueli Endowed Chair in the Susan Samueli Integrative Health Institute and professor in the Department of Anesthesiology and Perioperative Care in the School of Medicine at the University of California, Irvine. His background is in basic science and clinical research in alternative medicine. He received his BS degree in genetics from Purdue University in 1992 and his PhD in molecular and cell biology from the University of California, Berkeley, in 1997. Following his graduate work, he completed a postdoctoral fellowship at National Institutes of Health. He is a graduate of the Maryland Institute of Traditional Chinese Medicine and has received an MS degree in clinical research design and statistical analysis at the University of Michigan. Harris is currently investigating mechanisms of chronic pain and its treatment with acupuncture and shamanism. His recent investigations have focused on the role of brain neurotransmitters and brain network behavior in chronic pain. He was a member of the National Advisory Council for National Institutes of Health/National Center for Complementary and Integrative Health and is a current co-president for the Society for Acupuncture Research.

Allen Heinemann, PhD, MA, (Planning Committee Chair) is a professor of physical medicine and rehabilitation at Northwestern University's Feinberg School of Medicine and director of the Center for Rehabilitation Outcomes Research at the Shirley Ryan AbilityLab. His research focuses on patient-reported outcomes and evaluating medical and vocational rehabilitation services. He led the development of the Rehabilitation Measures Database, an online resource for outcome instrument reviews. A diplomate in rehabilitation psychology, he is a fellow and past president of the American Congress of Rehabilitation Medicine (ACRM) and a fellow of the American Psychological Association (APA). Dr. Heinemann co-edits the *Archives of Physical Medicine and Rehabilitation* and serves on editorial boards of *Rehabilitation Psychology* and the *Journal of Head Trauma Rehabilitation*. As an author of more than 500 publications, he co-directs the Integrated Post-Doctoral Fellowship in Health Services and Outcomes Research at Northwestern. He has received the Distinguished Career Award from APA's Rehabilitation Psychology division and the Gold Key Award from ACRM. He completed his PhD in psychology at the University of Kansas and currently serves on the National Academies of Sciences, Engineering, and Medicine Standing Committee of Medical and Vocational Experts for the Social Security Administration's Disability Programs.

Juan M. Hincapie-Castillo, PharmD, MS, PhD, (Planning Committee Member) is an assistant professor of epidemiology at the University of North Carolina (UNC) at Chapel Hill. Prior to joining UNC, he was an assistant professor of pharmaceutical outcomes and policy at the University of Florida. His research is at the intersection of legal and pharmacoepidemiology, where he leverages large real-world data sources to evaluate and promote evidence-based policymaking. His primary focus is on improving prescribing policies and the provision of equitable pain management and safe psychotropic medication use. Dr. Hincapie-Castillo is a consultant for the Food and Drug Administration's Drug Safety and Risk Management Advisory Committee. In 2021, he was appointed as a research fellow for the Center for Public Health Law Research at Temple University. He is a graduate from the University of Florida College of Pharmacy where he received the degrees of Doctor of Pharmacy, Master of Science in Pharmaceutical Sciences, and PhD with a concentration in pharmacoepidemiology. He is the recipient of the 2020 New Investigator Award from the American Association of Colleges of Pharmacy and the 2020 Emerging Leader Award from the International Society for Pharmacoepidemiology. He currently serves as president of the board of directors and member of the Science & Policy Advisory Board for the National Pain Advocacy Center.

Kim Dupree Jones, PhD, RN, FNP, FAAN, (Planning Committee Member) is a professor and associate dean for academic advancement at Emory University. Formerly, she was dean and professor at Linfield University's School of Nursing and a professor at Oregon Health & Science University. Her research focuses on fibromyalgia, a chronic pain condition that primarily affects women. She has led 60 studies funded by the National Institutes of Health, Department of Defense, and foundations, resulting in more than 130 publications. Her work is referenced in major medical texts, including *Cecil's Textbook of Medicine* and *Kelly's Textbook of Rheumatology.* Dr. Jones has extensive clinical experience as a family nurse practitioner and advanced her expertise with postdoctoral training in neuroendocrine physiology. In Oregon, she was appointed by the legislature to create pain management courses for prescribers and successfully advocated for fibromyalgia disability coverage under Medicaid. She is recognized as a fellow of the American Academy of Nursing and was inducted into the Sigma International Nurse Researcher Hall of Fame for her contributions to the field. Dr. Jones received her PhD in nursing from Oregon Health & Science University.

Ming-Chih Jeffrey Kao, PhD, MD, is faculty at Stanford Pain Management Center. He studied molecular biology and psychology at the University of California, Berkeley. At Harvard University, he earned a PhD in biostatistics after developing statistical methods in genomics and computational biology. He then pursued medical training at the University of Michigan and completed his internship at Yale New Haven Hospital. Kao came to Stanford University in 2012 where he completed his residency at Stanford's Division of Physical Medicine and Rehabilitation and completed a fellowship at Stanford's Division of Pain Management. He is board certified in pain medicine and physical medicine and rehabilitation. Kao is the author of more than 30 scientific journal articles, ranging from genetics, genomics, proteomics, combinatorial chemistry, artificial intelligence, oncology, epidemiology, rehabilitation, and pain. His mission is to offer all of his patients comprehensive interdisciplinary pain care, leveraging the full extent of what is known in state-of-the-art pain medicine.

Sean Mackey, MD, PhD, (Planning Committee Member) is Redlich Professor of Anesthesiology, Perioperative, and Pain Medicine; chief of the Division of Pain Medicine; and director of the Stanford Systems Neuroscience and Pain Lab at Stanford University. He has served as principal investigator on multiple National Institutes of Health (NIH) and Food and Drug Administration grants to better understand the mechanisms of pain and translate that knowledge into safe and effective therapies. In 2024 Dr. Mackey received the International Pelvic Pain Society James E. Carter Memorial Award and the Foundation for Anesthesia Education and Research-Helrich Lecture Award for his contributions to pain, neuroscience, and outcomes research. Past awards include American Academy of Pain Medicine's Founders Award; Robert G. Addison, MD Award; Presidential Commendation; Distinguished Service Award; American Pain Society's Wilbert E. Fordyce Clinical Investigator Award; and the NIH Director's Award for his leadership role on National Pain Strategy (NPS). He received his BSE and MSE in bioengineering from University of Pennsylvania and his PhD in electrical and computer engineering, as well as his MD from University of Arizona. He completed his residency and pain medicine fellowship at Stanford University. Dr. Mackey was co-author of the Institutes of Medicine's report *Relieving Pain in America*. He was co-chair of the Health and Human Services/NIH NPS, as well as vice chair for the Committee on Temporomandibular Disorders for National Academies of Sciences, Engineering, and Medicine/NIH.

Tom Norris is a veteran of the U.S. Air Force who has lived with chronic pain for nearly four decades following treatment for testicular cancer. He brings a deeply personal and sustained commitment to chronic pain advocacy, combining his lived experience with national-level engagement on research and policy. Norris currently facilitates multiple peer-led chronic pain support groups through the American Chronic Pain Association and other networks, creating welcoming spaces for individuals navigating life with chronic pain. As a patient advisor, he actively contributes to clinical trials and guideline development initiatives, championing meaningful patient engagement across research design, implementation, and dissemination. Norris's advocacy spans collaborations with organizations such as the U.S. Pain Foundation, National Institutes of Health-funded initiatives, and federal programs that seek to center patient voices—especially in the context of Social Security disability evaluations and access to comprehensive, multidisciplinary care.

Tonya Palermo, PhD, is professor and vice chair for research, Department of Anesthesiology and Pain Medicine at University of Washington, with adjunct appointments in pediatrics and psychiatry. She holds the Hughes M. and Katherine Blake Endowed Professorship in Health Psychology. Palermo serves as interim director of the Center for Child Health, Behavior and Development at Seattle Children's Research Institute, where she directs the Pediatric Pain and Sleep Innovations Lab. Her National Institutes of Health-funded research focuses on innovative psychological treatments for managing and preventing chronic pain in children, adolescents, and young adults. Palermo has published more than 350 articles and two books on cognitive behavioral therapy for pediatric chronic pain. Palermo is the editor in chief for the *Journal of Pain*. She is active in training clinician-scientists at the postdoctoral and faculty level and directs a T32 post-doctoral training program in anesthesiology research.

Kemly Philip, MD, PhD, MBE, is an assistant professor and division chief of musculoskeletal medicine and interventional pain in the Department of Physical Medicine and Rehabilitation at McGovern Medical School at UTHealth. Philip is a double-board-certified interventional pain special-ist focusing on management of spine and musculoskeletal disorders and electrodiagnostic medicine. Philip takes the time to develop a comprehen-sive, customized, and cutting-edge treatment plan for each patient with the goal of maximizing their function and quality of life with nonsurgical inter-ventions. She uses a multifaceted approach to pain management, includ-ing focused rehabilitation, diagnostic testing, and targeted, image-guided interventions. Philip received her Bachelor of Science in bioengineering and master of bioengineering from Rice University, followed by her MD/PhD through the Medical Scientist Training Program at the University of Texas MD Anderson Cancer Center UTHealth Graduate School of Biomedical Sciences and McGovern Medical School. She next completed her physi-cal medicine and rehabilitation residency at McGovern Medical School at UTHealth, where she served as academic chief resident from 2020 to 2021. She went on to complete her fellowship in pain medicine at the University of Colorado in Aurora before joining the esteemed faculty at McGovern Medical School. Philip is committed to undergraduate and graduate medi-cal education through her involvement in bedside teaching, lectures, and curriculum design, supporting the next generation of physicians in the management of chronic disability and neuromuscular and musculoskeletal disorders. Ultimately, as an interventional pain physician-scientist, she hopes to translate her background in bioengineering and research to create novel diagnostic and therapeutic treatments for patients suffering with pain. Philip is an active member of the Spine Intervention Society and American Academy of Physical Medicine and Rehabilitation.

Jaime Sanders is the author of the award-winning blog *The Migraine Diva* and the book *More Than Migraine: A Journey Through Pain, Advo-cacy, and Hope*. She is a participant with the Coalition for Headache and Migraine Patients, with whom she worked to create an issue brief on disparities in headache and served as part of the leadership of the Disparities in Headache Advisory Council. Sanders is a stakeholder with the Headache and Migraine Policy Forum, worked with the Society for Women's Health Research Interdisciplinary Migraine Network, sits on the Patient Leadership Council with the National Headache Foundation, and served on HealthyWomen's Chronic Pain Advisory Council. She has lived with migraine since the age of two and has been chronic and intractable for the last 18 years. Through her advocacy work and blog, Sanders's mission is to make a very invisible disease visible to the rest of the world and validate the real pain of millions.

Nathaniel "Nat" M. Schuster, MD, is a pain and headache neurologist and is professor and medical director at the University of California, San Diego Center for Pain Management. He serves on the board of directors of the American Academy of Pain Medicine, as senior vice president of the World Headache Society, as the vice chair of the Guidelines Committee for the International Pain and Spine Intervention Society. He has received the American Headache Society's Harold G. Wolff Award, the American Academy of Pain Medicine's Rollin "Mac" Gallagher Award, the International Pain and Spine Intervention Society's Outstanding Volunteer Award, and the Migraine Research Foundation's Impact Award. He is section editor for the Neuropathic Pain section for the journal *Pain Medicine*. He graduated from University of Michigan Medical School and completed a neurology residency at University of California, Los Angeles, headache fellowship at Montefiore Headache Center, and pain fellowship at Massachusetts General Hospital. He conducted the first placebo-controlled trial of cannabinoids for acute migraine and his ongoing research includes clinical trials studying treatments for headache and neuropathic pain.

Laura Simons, PhD, is a professor in the Department of Anesthesiology, Perioperative, and Pain Medicine at Stanford University Medical School and an attending psychologist at the pediatric pain management clinic at Stanford Children's Health. Simons is a committed researcher and clinician with a focus on psychological assessment and development of treatment interventions to improve the lives of youth with chronic pain. Before joining Stanford in 2016, she was an attending psychologist and associate professor at Boston Children's Hospital and Harvard Medical School. Over the decade she spent at Boston Children's Hospital she worked in the chronic pain clinic, pediatric headache program, and pediatric pain rehabilitation center.

Konstantin Slavin, MD, FAANS, is professor, chief of section, and fellowship director for Stereotactic and Functional Neurosurgery in the Department of

Neurosurgery at the University of Illinois Chicago (UIC). Slavin graduated from medical school in Baku, Azerbaijan, in the Soviet Union and completed his neurosurgery residency in Moscow. He then completed his second neurosurgery residency at UIC and a fellowship in functional and stereotactic neurosurgery at Oregon Health & Science University in Portland. Slavin is the current president of the International Neuromodulation Society, immediate past president of the World Society for Stereotactic and Functional Neurosurgery, and past president of the American Society for Stereotactic and Functional Neurosurgery. Slavin is published in many books and peer-reviewed journals and is an associate editor or editorial board member for a number of publications, including *Neuromodulation, Neurosurgery, Brain Sciences, Stereotactic and Functional Neurosurgery,* and *Acta Neurochirurgica*; he is the editor in chief of *Progress in Neurological Surgery.* His first book *Peripheral Nerve Stimulation* was published in 2011; another book, co-edited with Sam Eljamel, *Neurostimulation: Practice and Principles,* came out in 2013; a third, *Stimulation of Peripheral Nervous System: The Neuromodulation Frontier,* was released in 2015. His most recent book, *Neuromodulation for Facial Pain,* came out in 2021.

Christopher J. Standaert, MD, (Planning Committee Member) is a physiatrist and is board certified in physical medicine and rehabilitation and electrodiagnostic medicine. He is an associate professor in the Department of Physical Medicine and Rehabilitation Services at the University of Pittsburgh School of Medicine. He is also the vice chair of outpatient services and the director of Value-Based Fellowship in Spine and Musculoskeletal Medicine at the University of Pittsburgh Medical Center. Dr. Standaert specializes in the non-operative care of spine, joint, and neuromusculoskeletal disorders. He has worked extensively on health policy issues at state and national governmental levels as well as for multiple professional medical associations and hospital systems. His research interests include non-operative spine care, spinal injections, and health policy. Dr. Standaert received his medical degree from Harvard Medical School and completed his residency at the University of Washington, followed by his fellowship at Pioneer Spine and Sports Physicians. He currently serves on the National Academies of Sciences, Engineering, and Medicine Standing Committee of Medical and Vocational Experts for the Social Security Administration's Disability Programs.

Sebastian Tong, MD, MPH, (National Academy of Medicine Fellow) is a family physician, addiction medicine specialist, and health services researcher. He is an assistant professor in the Department of Family Medicine at the University of Washington. He also serves as the associate director of the Washington, Wyoming, Alaska, Montana, and Idaho region Practice and Research Network, a practice-based research network of more than

120 practices. He practices primary care at Harborview Family Medicine Center, a hospital-based safety-net clinic. Dr. Tong's research focuses on access to and implementation of evidence-based practices in primary care. He has a particular interest in chronic pain, substance use disorder, loneliness, and integrated behavioral health. He has received research funding for his work from the National Institutes of Health, the Agency for Healthcare Research and Quality, the American Board of Family Medicine Foundation, and the American Academy of Family Physicians Foundation. Dr. Tong is of the 2023–2025 National Academy of Medicine James C. Puffer/American Board of Family Medicine Fellows. In this capacity, he serves on the Standing Committee on Primary Care. Dr. Tong received his MD from Boston University School of Medicine and his MPH in health care management and policy from Harvard School of Public Health. He completed his family medicine training at Lawrence Family Medicine Residency in Lawrence, Massachusetts. He is certified by the American Board of Family Medicine and the American Board of Preventive Medicine in addiction medicine.

Carole Tucker, PT, PhD, is the associate dean of research, School of Health Professions, University of Texas Medical Branch (UTMB), Galveston. She also serves as director of the UTMB Center for Health Promotion, Performance and Rehabilitation Research, as well as chair of the Department of Physical Therapy and Rehabilitation Sciences. Her education includes degrees in physical therapy, electrical engineering, and exercise science. Her research interests include rehabilitation, digital health technology, health informatics, measurement science, patient-reported health outcomes, application of artificial intelligence and machine learning in health care, and lifespan health, particularly in pediatrics. She has received funding for her research from the National Institutes of Health, National Science Foundation, and Department of Defense and serves on several editorial boards.

Christin Veasley, BS, is a nationally recognized advocate in the field of pain research, fueled by her own journey with chronic pain following a near-fatal accident in her teens. With a science background and a deep personal connection to the cause, she has spent her life fostering the advancement of rigorous pain science and ensuring that research translates into meaningful, lasting change for those living with pain. Veasley has been a passionate and effective voice at the federal level—raising awareness of chronic pain's widespread impact, advocating for an increased investment in pain science, and championing the essential role and inclusion of patients as equal partners in science. She holds numerous advisory roles in federal initiatives, academic studies, and collaborative public–private partnerships focused on improving pain research, care, education, and engagement. In 2009 Veasley cofounded the Chronic Pain Research Alliance (CPRA)—the only advocacy initiative dedicated to advancing research on chronic overlapping pain conditions. Through strategic partnerships, the CPRA promotes high-quality research, clinician and patient education, and the development of safe and effective treatments, as well as a whole-person model of care. She is cochair of the National Institutes of Health's (NIH's) ENGAGE Working Group, tasked with developing the first-ever agency-wide framework for integrating patients and the public in all NIH-funded clinical research. As a trusted voice in the field, Veasley has authored numerous scientific, policy, and educational publications, and is a sought-after speaker. Her work bridges the gap between science, policy, and the lived experience to improve outcomes for people with pain.

V. G. Vinod Vydiswaran, PhD, is an associate professor of learning health sciences and associate professor of information at University of Michigan. His research focuses on health care research involving natural language processing and artificial intelligence over clinical documentation, biomedical literature, and health-related social media. His current research encompasses developing and evaluating novel natural language processing and artificial intelligence approaches including large language models, neural and federated networks, information extraction pipelines, and social determinants of health to address various health informatics challenges. Vydiswaran mentors graduate students from the Medical School and the School of Information, as well as postdoctoral researchers and undergraduate students.

Peter Wayne, PhD, is an associate professor of medicine at Harvard Medical School and Brigham and Women's Hospital. He is the director of research for the Osher Center for Integrative Medicine and currently serves as interim center director. The primary focus of Wayne's research is evaluating how mind-body and related complementary and integrative medicine practices clinically impact chronic health conditions and understanding the physiological and psychological mechanisms underlying observed therapeutic effects. He has served as a principal or co-investigator on more than 25 National Institutes of Health-funded studies. He has been involved in the design, conduct, analysis, and interpretation of clinical trials evaluating the safety and efficacy of tai chi exercise for balance disorders, heart failure, chronic obstructive pulmonary disease, osteoporosis, and depression, and trials evaluating acupuncture for stroke-related paralysis, hypertension, endometriosis, and chemoradiation-related immune and swallowing side effects in cancer patients. Wayne is actively involved in the teaching and training of students and fellows in integrative medicine research. He serves as associate director for the National Institutes of Health-funded Harvard Medical School Research Fellowship in Complementary and Integrative Medicine.

His commitment to mentoring is reflected in his being awarded a National Institutes of Health K24 mid-career mentoring award.

Anna Williams, BEd, (Planning Commitee Member) serves as the vice president for Clusterbusters, a nonprofit serving patients and caregivers of those experiencing cluster headaches. She is on the Programming Committee for the Alliance for Headache Disorders Advocacy/The Headache Alliance (AHDA/THA) working to provide education in the headache space as well as plan their advocacy event Headache on the Hill. While Williams is an advocate, she is a patient first, who experiences cluster headache, migraine, trigeminal neuralgia, and a few other chronic pain conditions. She is a patient opinion leader with Coalition for Headache and Migraine Patients (CHAMP) working with leading organizations to best elevate headache patient experience. She has undergone training programs with CHAMP, AHDA/THA, and Miles for Migraine.

Anna Wilson, PhD, is a professor of pediatrics at Oregon Health & Science University (OHSU). Dr. Wilson is a clinical psychologist who provides assessment and treatment for children and adolescents with chronic pain as part of OHSU's multidisciplinary Pediatric Pain Management Center. As a principal investigator in the Advancing Research in Pediatric Pain Lab, she studies acute and chronic pain conditions in children and in parents, with the goal of identifying psychosocial, intergenerational, and behavioral targets for the prevention of chronic pain and related conditions. Her work has been supported by the National Institutes of Health, the American Pain Society, and the Medical Research Foundation of Oregon. She co-authored *When Children Feel Pain*, a book about the history and science of the field of pediatric pain told through the lens of patient and researcher experiences.

Anna Woodbury, MD, founded the Division for Pain Management at the Veterans Affairs Health Care System (VAHCS) in Atlanta and serves as the associate vice chair of research for the Department of Anesthesiology at Emory University. She is double-board-certified in anesthesiology and pain medicine and licensed to practice acupuncture. She is an associate professor of anesthesiology and pain management at Emory University School of Medicine and active in research at both Emory and VAHCS. She has been a member of the national Committee on Pain Medicine for the American Society of Anesthesiologists and has served on institutional and federal grant review committees including National Institutes of Health and VA study sections. She has presented nationally and written book chapters, articles, and clinical reviews on integrative medicine and neuromodulation, including applications for chronic pain management, anesthesia, and neuroprotection. She has also edited a *Pain Management Board Review* book. Her clinical expertise and research interests include the use of nonpharmacologic therapies for the management of pain, and she has a specific interest in understanding and treating myofascial pain syndromes.

Henry Xiang, MD, MPH, PhD, MBA, (Planning Committee Member) is a professor of pediatrics and epidemiology at the Ohio State University and director of the Center for Pediatric Trauma Research at Nationwide Children's Hospital. He also serves as co-director of the Pilot Translational and Clinical Studies Program at the Ohio State University's Clinical and Translational Science Institute. Dr. Xiang's research spans over 30 years, with a focus on trauma care, pediatric pain management, and the development of digital health solutions for chronic pain management and treatment. Dr. Xiang has pioneered the use of virtual reality for pain management, including its application in pediatric burn care, traumatic brain injury rehabilitation, and managing pain and anxiety during medical procedures. His research, continuously funded by the National Institutes of Health, Centers for Disease Control and Prevention, and Agency for Healthcare Research and Quality, has significantly advanced the understanding of how emerging technologies can alleviate pain, reduce opioid usage, and improve patient outcomes. Dr. Xiang's contributions are recognized globally, earning him accolades such as the Excellence in Science Award from the American Public Health Association (ICEHS), the Society for Advancement of Violence and Injury Research (SAVIR) Excellence in Violence and Injury Prevention Science Award, and the Kate Granger Compassionate Care Award. Dr. Xiang received his PhD from Colorado State University, his MD and MPH from Tongji Medical College, and his MBA from the Ohio State University.